D1831834

THE INDIAN MANUAL OF FIRST AID

Owing to the antiquity and rarity of this book, certain pages are regrettably absent, and readability is compromised due to the blurring of the original text. If you possess any insights regarding the availability of these missing sections, kindly inform us. Your assistance is crucial in ensuring the completion of this significant work for the benefit of future generations.

THE

INDIAN MANUAL

OF

FIRST AID

ROBERT J. BLACKHAM

GYAN

Published by

Gyan Publishing House
5, Ansari Road
Daryaganj, New Delhi-110002
Phone: 011-47034999, 9811692060
E-mail: books@gyanbooks.com

Distribution Network
gyanbooks.com
India, USA, Canada, UK, Australia

© Publisher

All rights reserved. No part of this work may be reproduced, stored, adapted, or transmitted in any form or by any means, electronic, mechanical, photocopying, micro-filming, recording or otherwise, or translated in any language, without the prior written permission of the copyright owner and the publisher.

ISBN: 978-93-7097-530-9 (HB)

First Published, 1916

2nd Impression 2025

Printed at: Gyan Press, Delhi.

The book is sold subject to the condition that it shall not, by way of trade or otherwise, be lent, resold, hired out, or otherwise circulated without the prior publisher's written consent.

THE INDIAN MANUAL OF FIRST AID
Author: ROBERT J. BLACKHAM

THE BONES AND ARTERIES OF THE BODY.

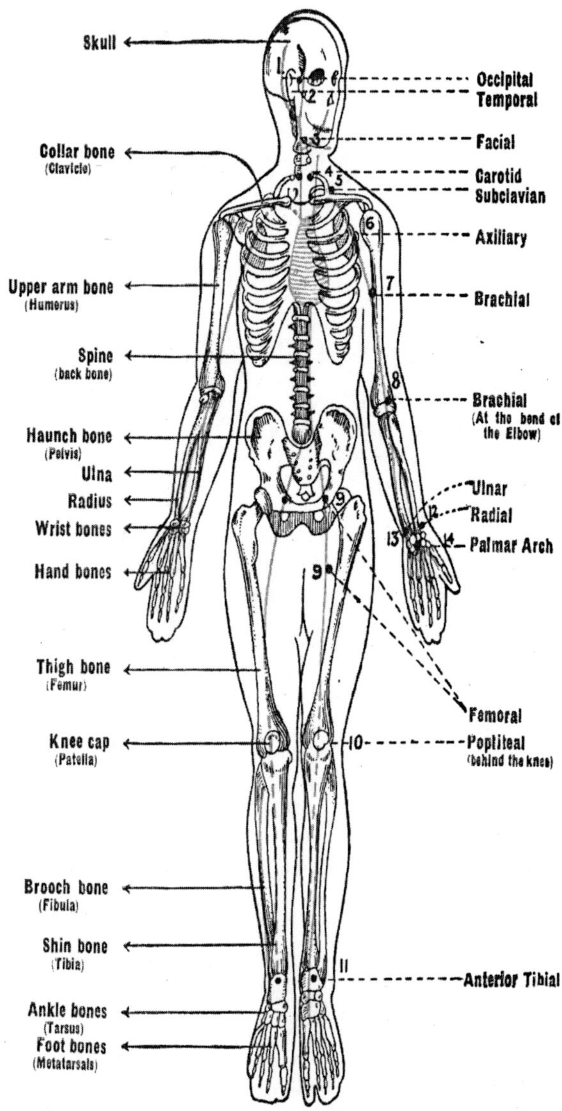

PRESSURE POINTS.

1. Back of head.
2. Front of head.
3. Face.
4. Neck.
5. Arm-pit pressure point.
6. Arm above elbow.
7. Arm above elbow.
8. Forearm.
9. For middle of ham.
10. Behind the Knee.
11. Ankle pressure point.
12. Wrist „

The black dots indicate the pressure points.

All Rights Reserved.]

THE INDIAN MANUAL OF FIRST AID

BY

COLONEL R. J. BLACKHAM, C.I.E.,
M.R.C.P.E., D.P.H. (LOND.), A.M.S.,
KNIGHT OF GRACE OF ST. JOHN,
KAISER-I-HIND MEDALLIST,
BARRISTER-AT-LAW,
ASST. COMMISSIONER, ST. JOHN AMB. BRIGADE,
ASST. DIRECTOR OF MEDICAL SERVICES OF A DIVISION,
BRITISH EXPEDITIONARY FORCE IN FRANCE.

SIXTEENTH EDITION.

(TWENTY-EIGHTH THOUSAND.)

Bombay:
G. CLARIDGE & CO.,
CAXTON HOUSE.
1916.

COMPANION VOLUMES

(BY THE SAME AUTHOR.)

THE INDIAN CATECHISM OF FIRST AID.
Second Edition. **Price :—Ten Annas.**

INDIAN HOME NURSING.
Fourth Edition. **Price :—One Rupee Four Annas.**

THE INDIAN CATECHISM OF HOME NURSING.
Price :—Twelve Annas.

TROPICAL HYGIENE.
(With The Hon'ble Surgeon-General Sir PARDEY LUKIS, K.C.S.I.)

Third Edition. **Price :—Three Rupees.**

THE PRIMER OF TROPICAL HYGIENE.
Third Edition. **Price :—One Rupee.**

INDIAN AMBULANCE TRAINING.
Price :—One Rupee.

SPECIMEN EXAMINATION PAPERS IN FIRST AID, HOME NURSING AND HYGIENE.
Second Edition. **Price :—Eight Annas.**

INDIAN HOUSEHOLD EMERGENCY CHART.
Price :—One Rupee Eight Annas.

INDIAN HOUSEHOLD REFERENCE CHART.
Price :—One Rupee Eight Annas.

Copies of the above are obtainable from
ALL BOOKSELLERS
OR
THE INDIAN STORES DEPOT.
St. John Ambulance Association,
P. BOX 353, BOMBAY.

PREFACE TO SIXTEENTH EDITION.

Fifteen editions having been exhausted in less than four years the publishers are justified in believing that their Manual has supplied a want amongst ambulance workers in India.

The student is strongly advised to use the *Indian Catechism of First Aid* in conjunction with this book when preparing for an examination or competition. He will find that every important point in each chapter is brought out in the form of question and answer in the Catechism

The *Indian Manual of First Aid* is the official text-book of the Indian Branch, S.J. A. A., and is the standard book for all ambulance competitions in India.

St. John Ambulance Association.

INDIAN BRANCH.

SYLLABUS OF INSTRUCTION

IN

FIRST AID TO THE INJURED.

FIRST LECTURE.

A. Preliminary remarks, objects of instruction, etc.

B. A brief description of the human skeleton, bones, joints, and the muscular system.

C. Signs, symptoms and treatment of fractures, dislocations, sprains and strains.

D. The triangular bandage and its application.

SECOND LECTURE.

A. The heart and blood vessels. The circulation of the blood.

B. The general direction of the main arteries, indicating the points where the circulation may be arrested by digital pressure or by the application of a tourniquet or by other means.

C. The difference between arterial, venous and capillary bleeding, and the various extemporary means of arresting it.

D. The triangular bandage and its application.

THIRD LECTURE.

A. A brief description of the nervous system.

B. First aid to persons suffering from shock or collapse after injury; injury to the brain, collapse from drink, epilepsy, fainting, hysteria, sunstroke, electric shock, effects of lightning, and convulsions in children.

C. First aid in cases of frost-bite, burns and scalds, injury by vitriol-throwing, wounds, bites of animals, and stings of insects.

D. What to do when the dress catches fire.

E. The triangular bandage and its application.

FOURTH LECTURE.

A. A brief description of the organs and mechan ism of respiration.

B. The immediate treatment of the apparently drowned, or otherwise suffocated; artificial respiration; treatment for choking.

C. First aid to those poisoned.

D. The immediate first aid treatment of injuries to the internal organs, and of those suffering from internal hæmorrhage.

E. Foreign bodies in the eye, ear and nose.

FIFTH LECTURE (FOR MALES ONLY.)

A. Improvised method of lifting and carrying the sick or injured.

B. Methods of lifting and carrying the sick or injured on stretchers.

C. The conveyance of such by rail or in country carts.

FIFTH LECTURE (FOR FEMALES ONLY.)

A. Preparation for reception of accident cases.

B. Means of lifting and carrying.

C. Preparation of bed.

D. Removing the clothes.

E. Preparations for surgeon.

NOTE FOR LECTURERS.

The subject-matter for the five official lectures of the Branch will be found as follows :—

Lecture I.—Chapters I, II, IV, V & VI.

Lecture II.—Chapters VII & VIII.

Lecture III.—Chapters IX, X & XI.

Lecture IV.—Chapters XII, XIII & XIV.

Lecture V.—(Males) Chapters XV & XVI.

Lecture V.—(Females) Chapter XVII.

Chapter III is required for the first four lectures.

SUMMARY OF CONTENTS.

CHAPTER I.

CHAPTER II.

CHAPTER III.

CHAPTER IV.

LIST OF ILLUSTRATIONS.

Litho.

*Denotes illustrations kindly lent by the Chief Secretary of the St. John Ambulance Association, London.

CHAPTER I.

THE PRINCIPLES OF FIRST AID.

FIRST Aid is a special branch of medical and surgical knowledge for the instruction of lay persons in the art of rendering temporary aid in accidents and in cases of sudden illness. The ambulance student is neither taught to be a nurse nor a quack doctor, but is simply and fully instructed in what he or she should do in the absence of skilled medical or surgical advice.

The principles which guide the First Aid student are seven in number, *viz.* :—

1. That his duty is to endeavour to obtain medical assistance and whilst waiting for the doctor to merely attend to actual emergencies. He is never to undertake the continued treatment of injuries or sickness.

2. That he must, if possible, promptly remove the cause of injuries or danger.

3. That where an injury is associated with hæmorrhage, he must first stop the bleeding.

4. That an injured part must be placed n as comfortable a position as possible.

5. That he must accustom himself to utilizing improvised material, as accidents generally happen when no material, such as splints and bandages, are at hand.

6. That an injured person must be given as much air as possible and kept warm or cool, as the case may be.

7. That he should endeavour to be :—

(*a*) *Observant*, that he may note the *causes* and *signs* of injury.

(*b*) *Tactful*, that he may without thoughtless questions learn the *symptoms* and *history* of the case—

(1) *Signs* are what may be perceived.

(2) *Symptoms* are what the patient can tell you.

(3) *History* means the circumstances attending the accident or sudden illness.

(*c*) *Resourceful*, that he may use to the best advantage whatever is at hand to prevent further damage and to assist Nature's efforts to repair the mischief already done.

(*d*) *Explicit*, that he may give clear instructions to the patient or the bystanders how best to assist him.

(*e*) *Discriminating*, that he may decide which of several injuries press most for treatment by himself, and what can best be left for the patient or the bystanders to do.

CHAPTER II.

THE HUMAN SKELETON.

THE human body is built up on a framework consisting of two hundred bones. The bones determine the general shape and proportions of the body, give attachment to the muscles, and form levers on which the muscles act to move the body or limbs from one position to another. They also form firm coverings for the protection of important organs.

It is unnecessary for the beginner at First Aid to learn or remember the names of all the bones. The following facts are all that it is necessary for him to know, but it is convenient for the senior Ambulance man to know the names of the principal bones and they are therefore given in brackets.

THE SKULL.

The bones of the head and face constitute the skull, which consists of a number of bones intimately joined together with the exception of the lower jaw which moves freely on a hinged joint.

The last named bone is frequently broken and presents special difficulties to the surgeon on account of having the lower teeth inserted in it.

When the other bones of the skull are broken, there is often great danger, as the skull contains the brain and the broken pieces of bone not infrequently press on its surface and produce unconsciousness and other symptoms (*vide* Table of Insensibility *p.* 98*a.*)

THE BONES OF THE BODY.

These are :—

1. The Back-bone or Spine.
2. The Breast-bone (or *Sternum*).
3. The Ribs.
4. The Pelvis consisting of two haunch bones, the rump bone and the tail bone.

1. The *back-bone* or *spine* consists of a number of bones joined together. Two of these bones which are situated in the neck are freely movable. The remainder are also capable of movement, but the

continuations of the spine known as the rump and tail bone are immovable.

Between the bones of the spine are discs of gristle or cartilage about a quarter of an inch thick.

The spine acts as a mainstay for the whole body, supports the head and transmits the weight of the upper part to the lower. The pads of gristle act as buffers to prevent shocks and jars being transmitted to the brain. They also serve to bind the bones together and convert them into a long flexible column.

The bones of the spine are so adapted as to form a long canal in which is enclosed a prolongation of the lower and back part of the brain which is known as the *spinal cord.*

The nerves which control the movements of the limbs originate from this portion of the nervous system and an injury of the spine usually means injury of the nerves of the limbs and consequent paralysis.

2. The *breast-bone* or *sternum* is a long flat dagger-shaped bone, the lower part of which consists of gristle or cartilage.

3. The *ribs* are twenty-four in number, twelve on each side. The upper seven are connected directly with the breast-bone in front and back-bone behind and are called *true ribs*. The next three pairs are each connected with the cartilage next above so that they are united to each other before they reach the sternum. The remaining two pairs are not connected in any way with the breast-bone. The five lowermost pairs are termed the *false ribs*: and of these the last two pairs are called free or *floating ribs*.

4. The *pelvis* is a large basin-shaped girdle which exists for the support and protection of some of the most important organs of the body. Its outer surface enters into the formation of the hip-joint and affords attachment for the muscles of the lower limbs.

It consists of :—

1. The Two Haunch Bones.
2. The Rump Bone.
3. The Tail Bone.

1. *The Haunch Bones.*—These are two large thick irregular shaped bones joined

in front but separated behind by the rump and tail bones. Each haunch bone has a large smooth inner surface which forms part of the side wall of the lower part of the belly. On the outer side of each is a deep, cup-shaped socket into which the head of the thigh bone fits to form the hip-joint.

2. *The Rump Bone.*—This is really a portion of the spine and is composed of five bones, separate in childhood but joined together in adult life.

3. *The Tail Bone.*—This is the rudimentary tail of man. It is a continuation of the rump bone and consists of four little bones, fused together into a cone shaped mass.

THE BONES OF THE UPPER LIMB.

These are :—

1. The Shoulder Blade (or *Scapula.*)
2. The Collar Bone (or *Clavicle.*)
3. The Upper Arm Bone (or *Humerus.*)
4. The Forearm Bones, (*Radius* on the outer side and *Ulna* on the inner side).

5. The Wrist (or *Carpal* Bones).
6. The Hand (or *Metacarpal* Bones and *Phalanges*).

1. *The Shoulder Blade* (*Scapula*).—This is a large flat triangular bone which lies on the ribs at the upper part of the back of the chest and has attached to it most of the muscles which move the arm. It has a strong broad process which forms a joint with the collar-bone. Owing to its free movement on the ribs it is seldom broken.

2. *The Collar Bone* (*Clavicle*).—This is a small bone shaped like a very open letter S. It forms joints with the breast-bone and the shoulder-blade. It is more often broken than any other bone in the body. It is so frequently broken in falls from horses that fracture of the collar-bone is often called "Jockey's Fracture."

3. *The Upper Arm Bone* (***Humerus***).—This is a large bone having at its upper end a rounded head, which works in a shallow socket in the shoulder-blade, and at its lower end a roller-shaped surface, which, with the bones of the forearm, forms the elbow-joint.

4. *The Forearm Bones.*—These are two in number. The outer one or *radius* extends from the thumb-side of the elbow to the thumb-side of the wrist. The inner one or *ulna* extends from the little finger side of the elbow to the little finger side of the wrist. At the upper end of the inner bone is a projection which forms the point of the elbow. There is a space between the two bones and the outer one has the power of rotating round the inner one.

When the palm of the hand points either upwards or downwards, these two bones are in close contact. When, however, the thumb points upwards they are far apart. This is an important point in dealing with fractures of the forearm as if the broken bones were put up in contact false joints and adhesions might occur.

5. *The Wrist Bones* (*Carpus*).—The wrist consists of eight little bones beautifully fitted together so as to facilitate the delicate movements of the wrist.

6. *The Hand Bones.*—These are arranged in two rows: (*a*) A row of five long metacarpal bones forming the frame work of the

palm, and (*b*) a row of small bones three for each finger and two for the thumb.

THE BONES OF THE LOWER LIMB.

These are :—

1. The Thigh Bone (or *Femur*).
2. The Knee Cap (or *Patella*).
3. The Leg Bones, (*Tibia* and *Fibula*).
4. The Foot Bones.

1. *The Thigh Bone* (*Femur*).—This is a long cylindrical bone, very liable to fracture. It is joined above by a ball-and-socket joint to the hip-bone and below by a hinge-joint to the shin-bone. It is the largest bone in the body.

2. *The Knee Cap* (*or Patella*).—This is a thick triangular bone situated in front of the knee-joint and resting on the lower part of the thigh bone. It protects the front of the joint, and increases the power of the muscles of the front of the thigh.

3. *The Leg Bones.*—These are two in number, *viz.* :—

(*a*) The Shin Bone or *Tibia* ; and (*b*) The Splint Bone or *Fibula.*

(*a*) *The Shin Bone* (*Tibia*).—This is placed at the front and inner side of the leg. It is the second longest bone in the body. Its upper end is large and supports the thigh bone forming with it and the knee-cap the knee-joint. A large portion of its inner surface is immediately beneath the skin. A stout prolongation on the inner side constitutes the inner support of the ankle joint.

(*b*) *The Splint Bone* (*Fibula*).—This is the smaller of the two bones of the leg and in proportion to its length the most slender bone in the skeleton. Its upper and lower ends are fixed to the outer side of the shin-bone thereby greatly increasing its strength; hence its name of *Splint Bone.*

4. *The Foot Bones.*—The construction of the foot is similar to that of the hand. The bones are arranged in three rows forming :—

(*a*) The Ankle; (*b*) The Sole of the Foot; and (*c*) The Toes.

(*a*) The hinder part or ankle is formed of seven short strong *tarsal* bones.

(*b*) The sole of the foot and instep is composed of a row of five longer metatarsal bones, and lastly—

(*c*) The toes are formed of small bones, three for each of the four outer toes and two for the great toe.

Joints and Ligaments.—A joint is formed where two or more bones work on each other. The ends of the bones where they touch one another are covered with a smooth gristle or cartilage, and are kept together by bands of binding material which permit movements only in certain directions thereby preventing the bones from slipping out of place. These bands are called *ligaments.* To enable the ends of the bones to glide smoothly over one another, joint oil, which is a material somewhat like white of egg, is provided.

The two principal kinds of joints are (*a*) the ball and socket, and (*b*) the hinge-joint.

(*a*) The ball-and-socket joint allows one of the bones to move freely in all directions as in the case of the shoulders and hip.

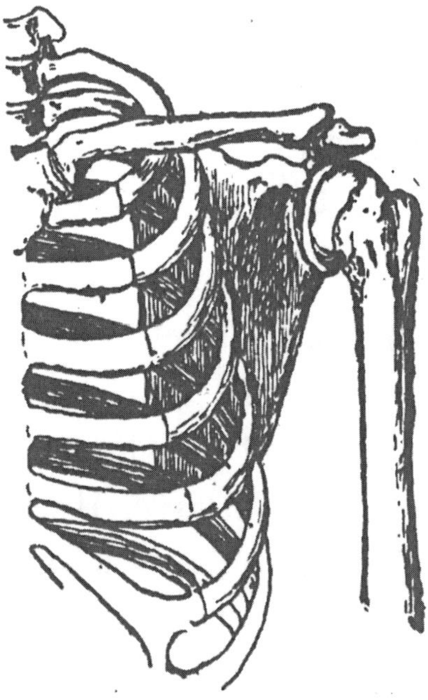

FIG. 2.

BALL-AND-SOCKET JOINT.
(SHOULDER).

(*b*) The hinge-joint as its name implies allows of movements up and down or backwards and forwards only and is seen in the elbow and knee.

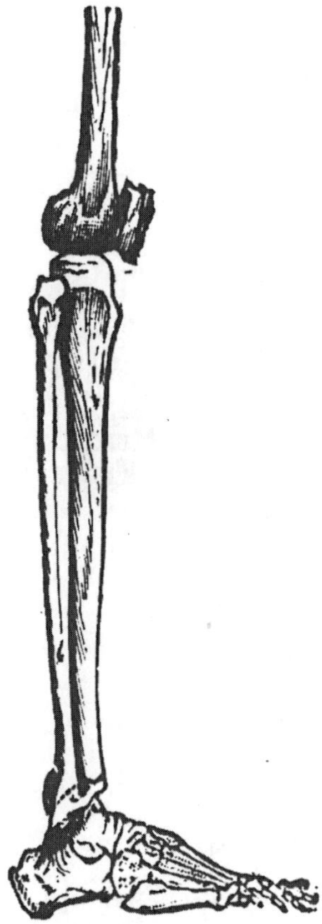

FIG. 3.

HINGE-JOINT—THE KNEE.

Muscles.—Flesh is the popular name for muscles. The lean portion of a piece of beef or mutton consists entirely of muscles.

The movements of the body are performed by muscles which are of two kinds, *viz.* :—(*a*) Voluntary, and (*b*) Involuntary.

(*a*) *Voluntary.*—Voluntary muscles are moved by the will of the individual. They are attached by their ends to bones, with generally a joint intervening with the result that when the muscle contracts, it draws together the bones to which its ends are attached. The

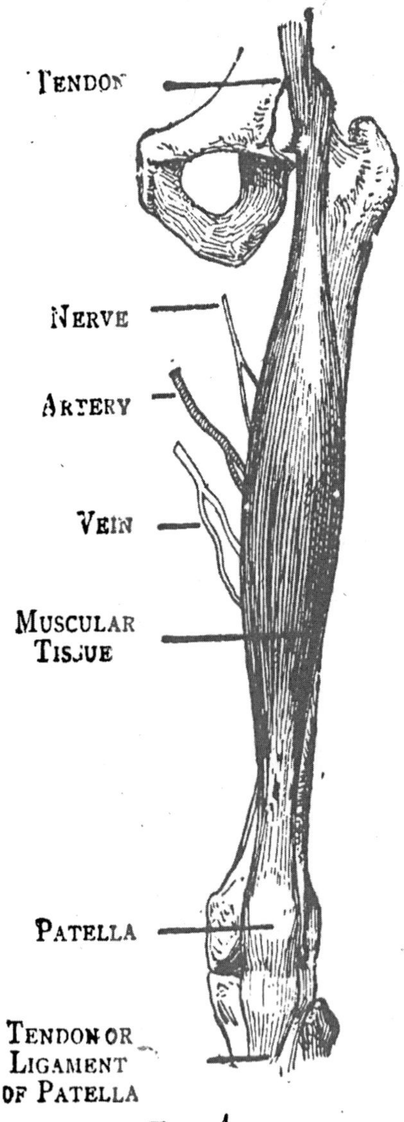

Fig 4.

contraction, for example, of the biceps muscle of the arm, one end of which is attached to the top of the shoulder-blade, the other to the forearm near the elbow-joint, bends the elbow and draws up the forearm. *Tendons* or *sinews* are the tough whitish cords by which the muscles are attached to the bones.

(*b*) *Involuntary.*—These are found chiefly in the blood vessels, stomach, intestines and other internal organs. They are not controlled by the will and are different in structure to voluntary muscles. They are controlled by the sympathetic nervous system (*see* Chapter XI). By the action of the involuntary muscles in the intestinal walls the food is passed along the bowels during the process of digestion. The heart is composed of involuntary muscles of a special kind.

CHAPTER III.

The Triangular Bandage.

The triangular bandage is particularly suitable for First Aid work, because :—

(1) Its application requires little practice.

(2) Its application is not associated with the risk of strangulation of tissues which may be produced by an improperly applied roller bandage.

(3) It can be improvised from a handkerchief or a square of cloth material a yard or perferably 38 inches in width, folded diagonally from corner to corner.

Of the three borders of the bandage the longest is called the *lower border*, and the two others the *side borders*. Of the three corners, the upper one, opposite the lower border, is called *the point* and the remaining corners *the ends*.

The Three Modes of Application.—The bandage is applied as (*a*) the whole-cloth " unfolded " or open bandage ; (*b*) broad-fold bandage ; (*c*) narrow-fold bandage.

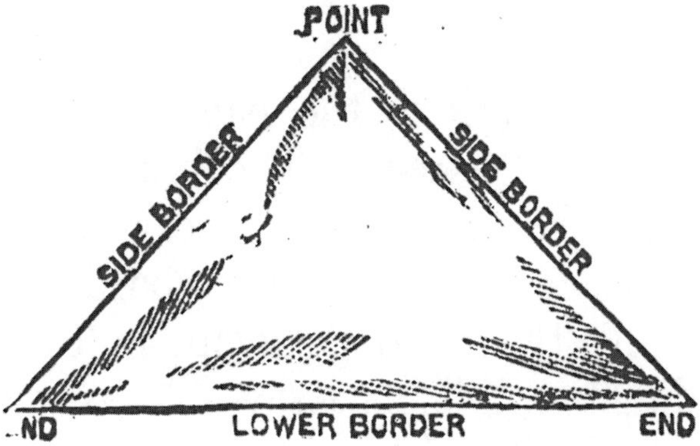

OPEN BANDAGE.

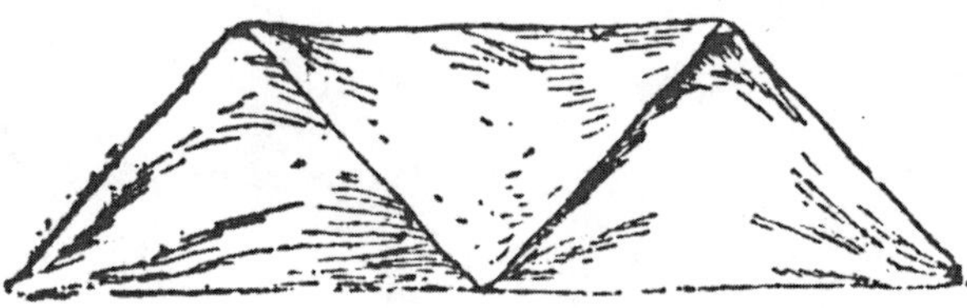

BANDAGE ONCE FOLDED.

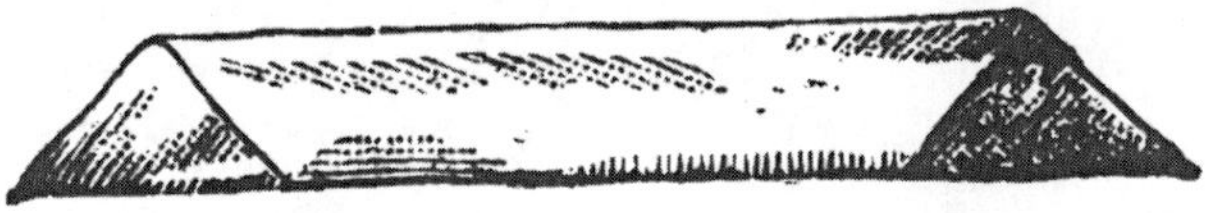

BROAD-FOLD BANDAGE.

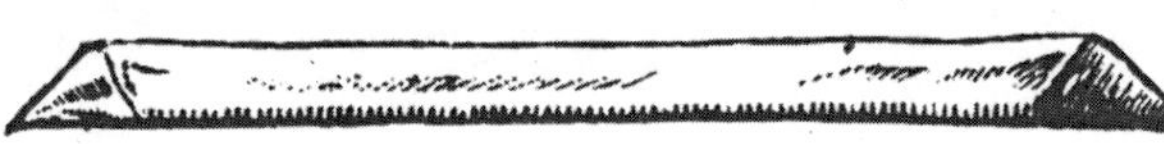

NARROW-FOLD BANDAGE.

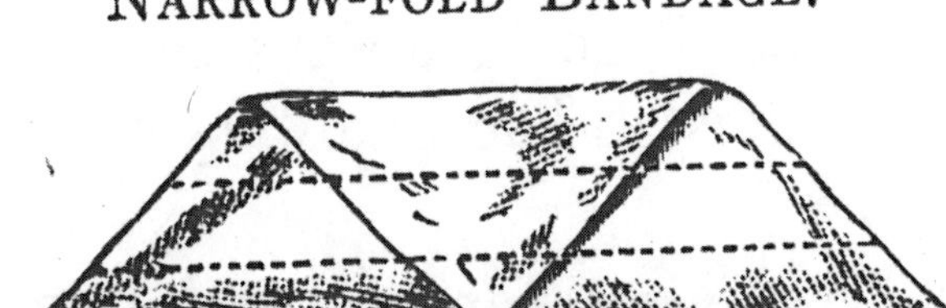

FIG. 5.—THE DOTTED LINES SHOW THE FOLDS OF THE MEDIUM BANDAGE.

The whole cloth is the bandage spread out to its full extent. The broad-fold is made from the whole-cloth by carrying the point to the centre of the lower border, and then folding the bandage again in the opposite direction. The narrow-fold is made by folding the broad-fold once lengthwise.

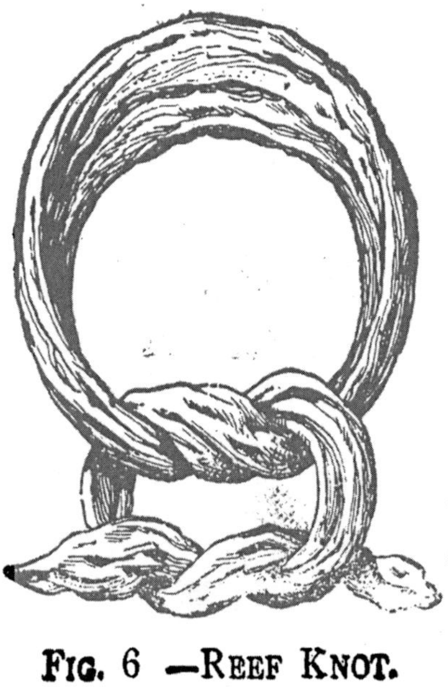

FIG. 6 —REEF KNOT.

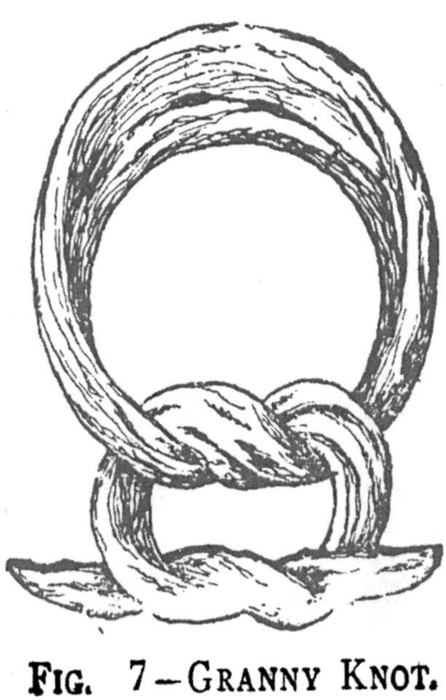

FIG. 7—GRANNY KNOT.

The bandage should always be put away carefully folded. The following is the be t method :—

Form a narrow bandage and bring the two ends together in the centre. Once more bring the extremities now formed together in the centre and then double the bandage upon itself. By this means the bandage is ready to be placed in the pocket.

Always tie the ends of bandages by *reef knots,* as *granny knots* are liable to slip and are hard to undo.

A *reef knot* is made as follows :—

Take one end of the bandage in the left hand and the other in the right, pass the left end in front of the right, and twist one end round the other in the usual method of making a knot, then pass the left hand behind the right, and finish the knot.

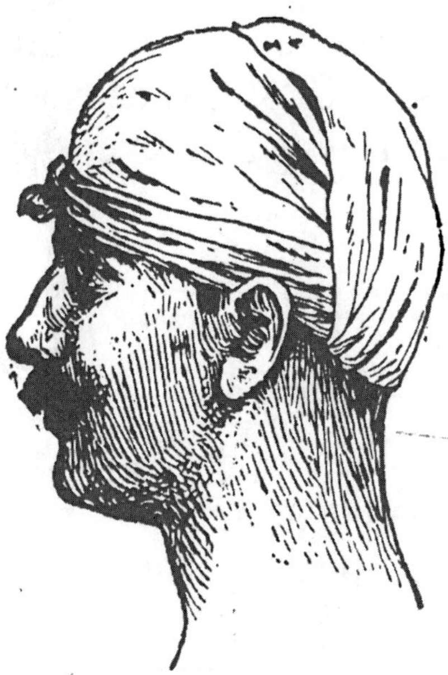

FIG. 8
HEAD BANDAGE.

THE HEAD BANDAGE.

(1) Fold a hem about $2\frac{1}{2}$ inches deep along the lower border. (2) Place the bandage on the

head, so that the hem lies squarely across the forehead and the point hangs down at the back. (3) Carry the two ends round the head above the ears. (4) Cross at the back. (5) Bring forward again and tie across the forehead.

The corner which hangs down is then drawn down tight, turned up, and secured on the top of the head with a safety pin.

The Jaw Bandage.

Apply a narrow bandage under the chin and then over the head. Cross the ends at angle of jaw and carry the long ends over the front of the chin and tie off.

The Shoulder Bandage.

See Fig. 9, *Page* 23.

(1) Apply an arm-sling. (2) Lay the centre of an open bandage on the top of the shoulder, point upwards, the lower border lying across the middle of the arm. (3) Fold the lower border, carry the ends round the arm, cross them. (4) Draw the point of the bandage under the

arm-sling, fold it back on itself. (5) Pin off over the shoulder.

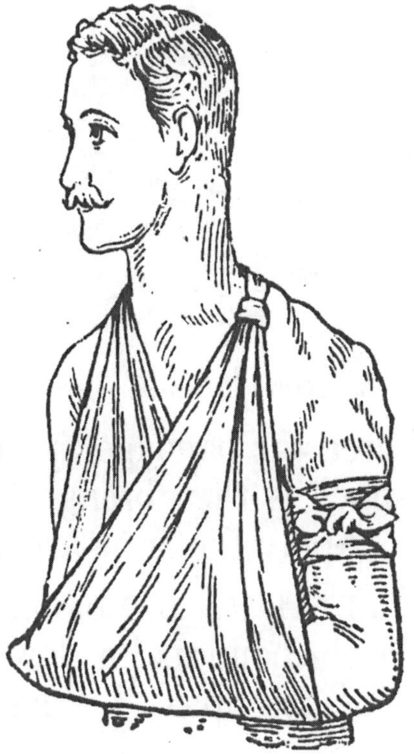

Fig. 9.—Shoulder Bandage.

THE ELBOW BANDAGE.

(1) Place the centre of an open triangular bandage over the back of the bent elbow, point upwards. (2) Turn in the lower border.

(3) Pass the ends round the forearm. (4) Cross them in front. (5) Pass up round the arm, cross behind, and knot off in

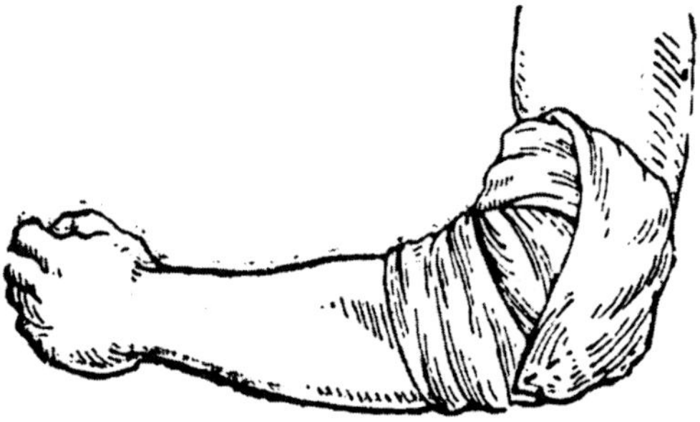

FIG. 10.

ELBOW BANDAGE.

front. Tighten the bandage by drawing on the point which is then brought down and pinned off. Apply the large arm-sling.

THE HAND BANDAGE.

(1) Place the hand, palm downward, on the centre of an open bandage, fingers

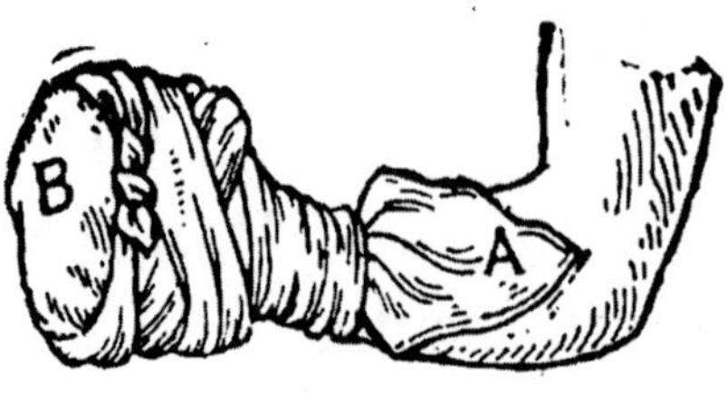

FIG. 11.

HAND BANDAGE (HAND CLOSED).

towards the point. (2) Bring the point over the back of the hand to the wrist. (3)

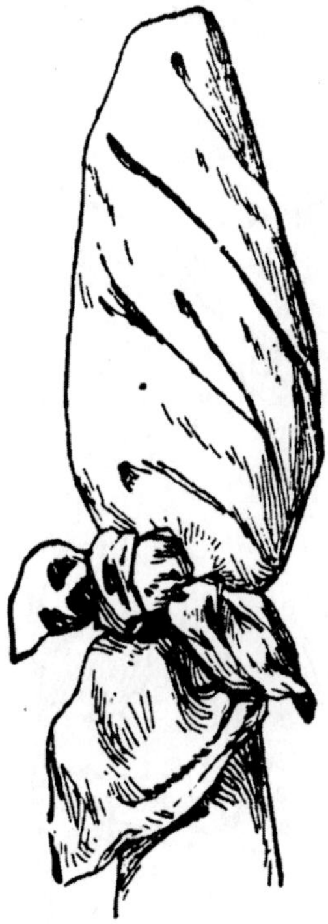

FIG. 12.

HAND BANDAGE (HAND OPEN.)

Pass the ends round the wrist crossing them over the point. (4) Fold the point towards the fingers, and cover it by another turn of the bandage round the wrist. (5) Knot off the ends in front of the wrist.

The Hip Bandage.

(1) Apply a narrow bandage round the waist, and knot off in front. (2) Take an

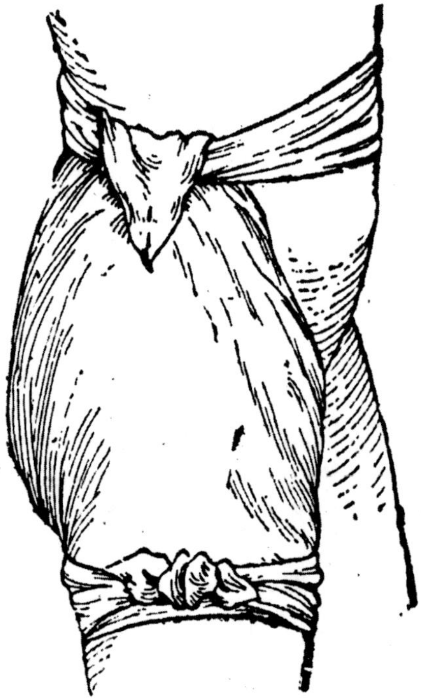

Fig 13.

Hip Bandage.

open bandage, place the centre over the hip, point upwards, the lower border, which should be folded in, lying across the thigh. (3) Pass the ends round the thigh, and knot off on the outer side. (4) Draw the point beneath the bandage round the waist. (5) Turn it down and pin off.

THE CHEST BANDAGE.

(1) Place the middle of the bandage over the dressing with the point over the shoulder on the same side. (2) Carry the ends round the body and tie them with one end longer than the other. (3) Tie the longer end to the point on the top of the shoulder.

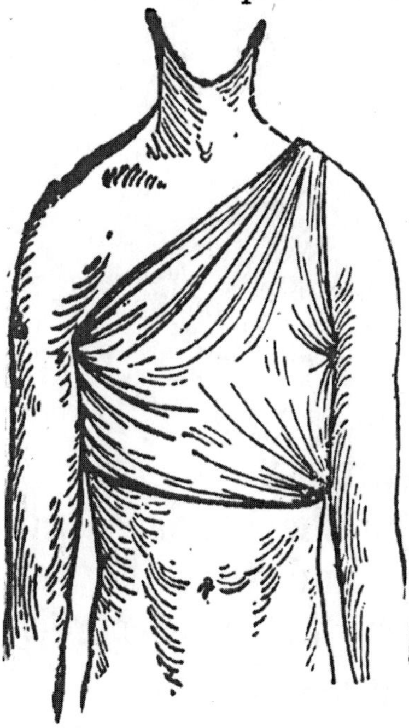

FIG. 14.

CHEST BANDAGE.
FRONT VIEW.

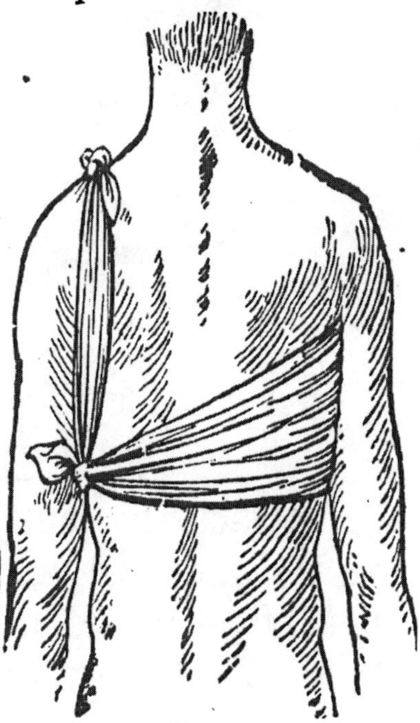

FIG. 15.

CHEST BANDAGE.
BACK VIEW.

THE FOOT BANDAGE.

1. Lay an open triangular bandage on the floor with its point away from patient.

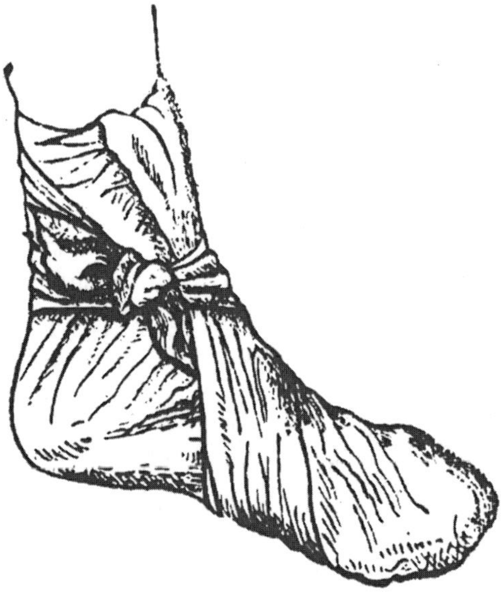

FIG. 16.
FOOT BANDAGE.

2. Place the foot on the bandage with toes towards the point and with the heel about four inches from the lower border. Draw the point over the instep.

3. Take up ends and cross them over the instep.

4. Carry them behind the ankle, cross again and bring them to the front of the

ankle and tie off.

5. Bring the point forward and pin it to fold of bandage in front of the ankle.

THE ARM SLINGS.

(1) *The Large Arm Sling* :—

1. Stand in front of patient.

2. Hold the point in one hand and one end in the other.

3. Lay the bandage on the front of the body, placing the point between the body and elbow of the injured side.

4. Carry one end over the shoulder of sound side, round the neck and over the shoulder of injured side.

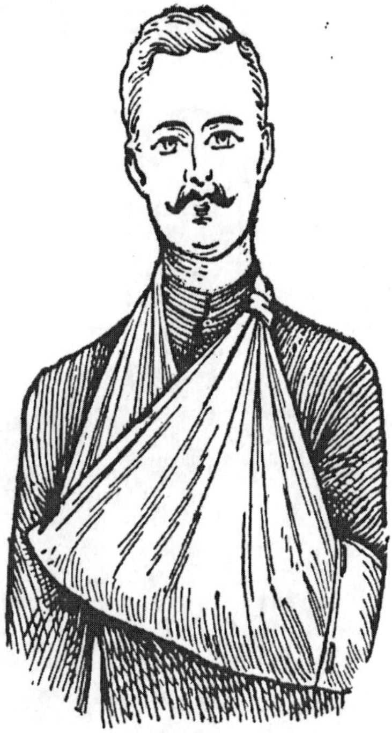

FIG. 17.

LARGE ARM SLING.

5. Bend the elbow and place the forearm and hand of the injured side on the bandage with the hand somewhat higher than the elbow.

6. Bring up the lower end of the bandage and tie it to the upper end.

7. Fold the point over the elbow and secure with a safety pin (*See* FIG. 17.)

(2) *The Small Arm Sling*:—

1. Fold a triangular bandage as the broad bandage.

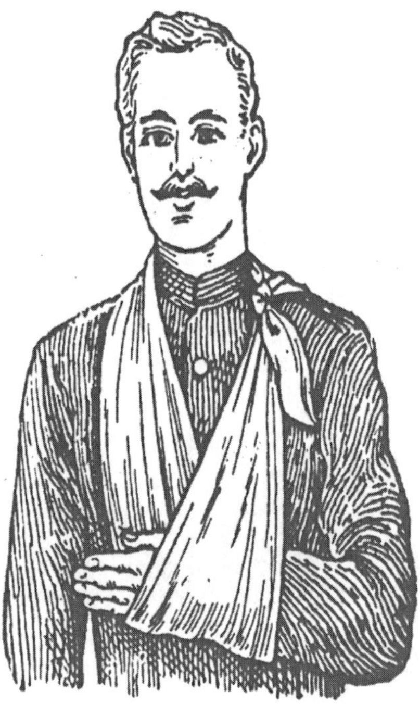

FIG. 18.

SMALL ARM SLING.

2. Lay one end across the sound shoulder and carry it round the back of the neck to the injured side.

3. Bend the elbow and, supporting the forearm, wrist and hand with the bandage, bring up the lower end and tie to upper end above the fold of the shoulder (*See* FIG. 18.)

The knot should not be placed at the back of the neck as in this position it is very inconvenient when the patient lies down.

CHAPTER IV.

Fractures and their General Treatment.

Bones are hard but brittle, and are frequently broken as the result of blows, falls, etc.

A fracture is simply a broken bone.

Fractures may be roughly divided into two kinds, namely, *simple* and *compound*. We call a fracture *simple* when the skin is not injured. We call it *compound* when it is accompanied by a wound, caused either by the same force which produced it or by the ends of the broken bone protruding through the skin.

In addition to these two chief classes there are the following :—

1. *Comminuted Fracture.*—In this variety the bone is crushed or broken into a number of pieces.

2. *Complicated Fracture.*—In this variety the jagged broken ends of the bone have injured an artery, vein or nerve.

Carelessness or unskilled movements of a broken limb may produce this variety.

3. *Green Stick Fracture.*—This occurs in children. The bones of children are not brittle and, therefore, are cracked or bent without being broken completely across by the same injuries which causes ordinary fractures in adults.

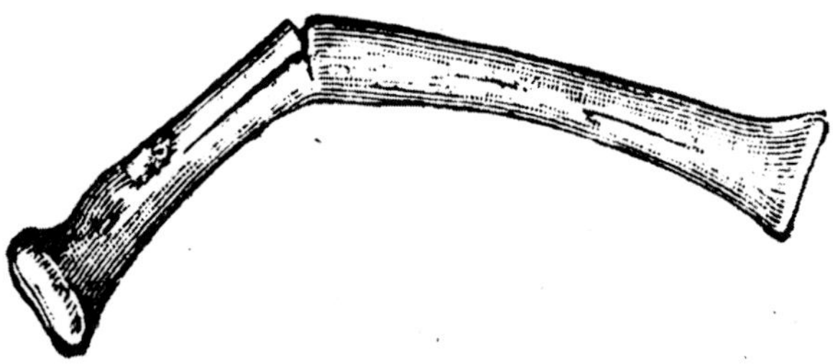

FIG. 19.

GREEN STICK FRACTURE.

4. *Impacted Fracture.*—This occurs when one broken end of the bone is forced into the other.

The Causes of Fracture :—1. *Direct Violence.*—A bone may be broken by a direct injury to it, such as occurs when the wheel of a carriage passes over a limb.

2. *Indirect Violence.*—A bone may be broken at some distance from the seat of an

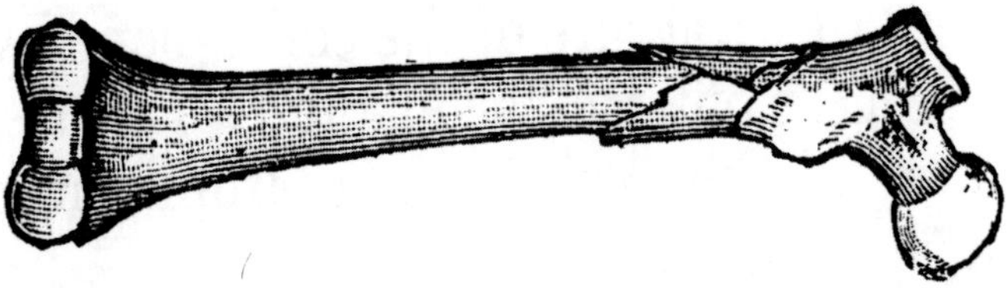

Comminuted Fracture of the upper end of the Right Thigh Bone.

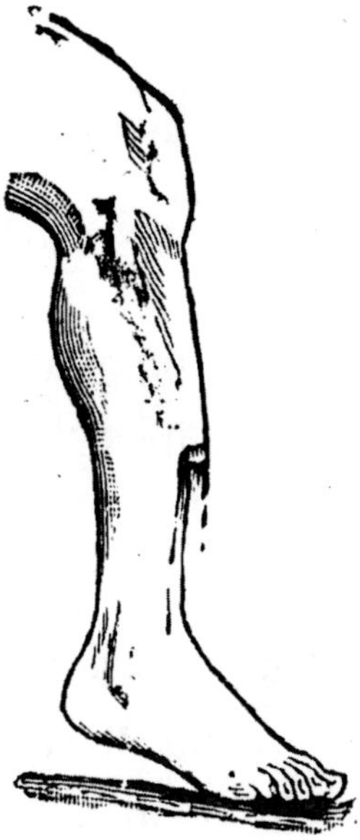

Compound Fracture of the Shin Bone.

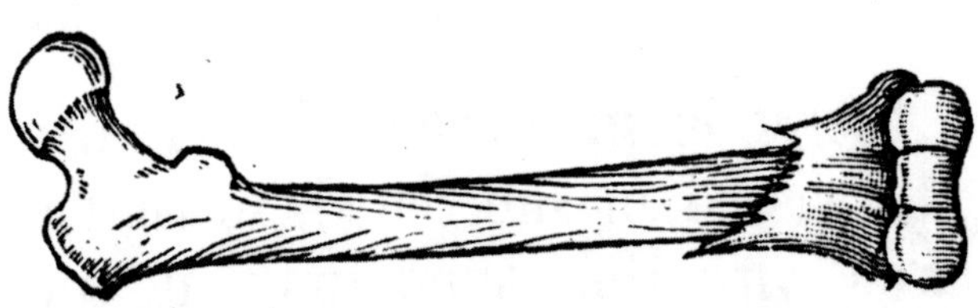

Fig. 20—Impacted Fracture of the lower end of the Right Thigh Bone.

injury through the transmission of the force applied, *e.g.*, fracture of the collar-bone by a fall upon the outstretched hand ; fracture of the base of the skull by a fall from a height upon the feet.

3. *Muscular Action.*—A bone may be snapped across by the sudden and violent action of a muscle, *e.g.*, the knee-cap may be fractured in jumping.

SIGNS AND SYMPTOMS OF FRACTURES.

1. *Pain.*—This is usually referred by the patient to the point at which the bone is broken.

2. *Uselessness of the Limb.*—The limb cannot be put to its proper use : for instance, when a leg is broken a man cannot stand upon it : when an arm is broken, the hand cannot be raised to the back of the head.

3. *Alteration in Shape.*—The limb may be bent, twisted, or shortened, so that when compared with the sound limb, it appears of an unnatural shape.

4. *Swelling.*—This is generally present. It is due to effusion of blood and contraction of the muscles which makes the bones override.

5. The patient usually complains of having felt or heard something give way with a snap.

The broken bone may be felt and if it is near the surface, as in the case of the collar-bone, it may be both seen and felt.

6. *Unnatural Mobility.*—This means that when the limb is handled (which should not be done unnecessarily) it gives way where, if sound, it would not be movable.

7. *Crepitus.*—When handled, there is generally a grating sensation, caused by the broken ends of the bone grating against one another. The ambulance man or women must, however, on no account try to obtain this sign lest the injury be aggravated in eliciting it.

Apparatus for Rendering First Aid in Fractures.

Surgeons use what are called *splints* in the treatment of fractures.

They are supports made of various materials adapted to fit the limbs and applied so as to render the joints above and below the injured part incapable of movement.

For First Aid purposes surgeon's splints are not available and temporary means of attaining a similar object must be devised from the following, or similar, articles :—

Lathis.
Pieces of Wood.
Walking sticks.
Umbrellas.
Whips.
Canes.
Guns.
Indian shoes.
Folded Newspapers.
Wine bottle covers, etc.

The surgeon keeps his splints in position with roller bandages; in rendering First Aid the ambulance man must utilise :—

Puggaries.
Handkerchiefs.
Straps, or any binding material which comes to his hand.

GENERAL RULES FOR TREATMENT OF FRACTURES.

1. Send for a doctor.
2. If there is any bleeding attend to it first and think of splints afterwards.
3. If in doubt as to what the injury is, treat as fracture.
4. Do not move the patient until he has been treated.
5. Prevent further injury by supporting the limb and applying rough and ready splints.
6. Reduce shock by keeping the patient warm.
7. If you consider that the backbone, pelvis or thigh is injured, keep the patient lying down.

Roughly speaking the time required for the healing of a fracture of the various bones is as follows :—

Rib, three weeks.
Collar Bone, four weeks.
Forearm Bones, five weeks.
Humerus, six weeks.
Leg Bones, seven weeks.
Thigh Bone, ten to twelve weeks.

CHAPTER V.

THE SPECIAL FRACTURES.

1. *Fracture of the Skull.*—This is frequently attended with unconsciousness, owing to injury to the brain. The roof of the skull may be fractured, or the injury may be seated at the base. Fracture of the latter may be suspected when there is bleeding from the ears, eyes, nose or mouth, or a watery discharge from one or both ears.

Treatment.—(1) Place the patient lying down with his head slightly raised. (2) Loosen the clothing round the neck and over the chest. (3) Do not give a stimulant. (4) Keep patient very quiet until medical assistance arrives. (5) Keep warm by every available means to prevent shock. (6) Arrange for transport on a stretcher.

2. *Fracture of Lower Jaw.*—This is a fairly common injury, all general signs of fracture are present and also the following *Special Signs*—

1. Irregularity of the teeth.
2. Bleeding from the gums.

All fractures of the lower jaw are compound.

Treatment :—

1. Press the lower against the upper jaw with palm of hand on the chin.

2. Place a narrow bandage with centre below the chin, carry over the head and cross just in front of and below the ear, bring long end over the front of the chin and then tie off.

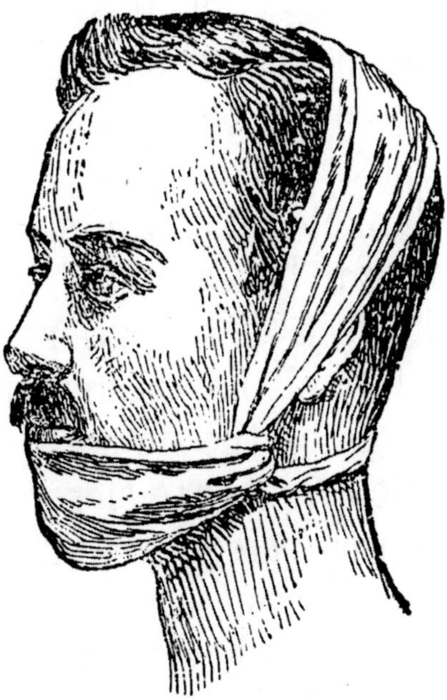

FIG. 21.
BANDAGE FOR FRACTURED LOWER JAW.

3. *Fracture of the Spine or Backbone.*—The Spine may be broken in any part of its extent. The special danger is injury to the spinal cord, which is followed by death or paralysis. The lower down the spine the fracture occurs the less the immediate danger to life.

Treatment.—Do not attempt to move the patient if medical assistance can be obtained, but, if no surgeon is available, proceed to render First Aid as follows :—

Place a blanket, horse cloth, or small durrie on the ground in a line with the patient's head. Two helpers kneeling one on each side gently pass the edge of the blanket under the shoulders and gradually drag it beneath the hips and legs as far as the feet. The patient must not be raised. After this has been done, two lathis must be placed on the support, one on each side, and rolled in quite close up to the body of the injured person, who is then slowly and with the utmost care carried by four people moving sideways to the nearest place of shelter, where he is kept absolutely quiet until the arrival of a surgeon. If lathis or poles are not available, helpers must seize the sides of the durrie or blanket and lift.

Instead of passing the durrie or blanket beneath the patient, his coat may be opened and rolled firmly up to the sides of the body. Two persons then take hold of the coat on either side and two others pass their hands beneath the hips and legs and the four acting together raise the patient and place him on a charpoy or stretcher. Keep the patient warm to avert shock.

4. *Fracture of the Ribs.*—Ribs may be broken by (*a*) direct violence, such as a blow or more usually, (*b*) indirect violence, such as pressure on the chest with the back against some unyielding support. In the latter case the ribs first bend and then break, often at some distance from the point where the pressure was applied. When the ribs are broken by direct violence, the fragments are driven inwards, and may puncture the lungs, liver, spleen, and diaphragm. When the injury is due to indirect violence, the internal organs are very rarely injured. The fifth to the eighth ribs are those most commonly broken.

Special Signs and Symptoms—

1. Severe pain on deep breathing or coughing.
2. If the hand is laid on seat of pain and a breath taken, crepitus may be felt.

Treatment—

Simple.—(1) Apply two broad folds of

puggaree or other material firmly round the chest. The centre of the first fold should be just above the painful part and the centre of the second fold just below it.

(2) Put the arm in a large arm sling.

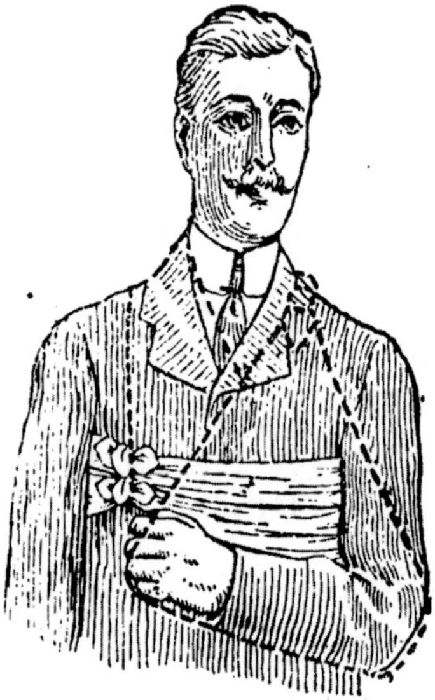

FIG. 22.
TREATMENT FOR FRACTURED RIBS.

COMPLICATED BY INTERNAL INJURY.

When a fracture of the ribs is complicated by injury of the lung the patient is collapsed and usually spits up blood. The treatment is as follows :—

(*a*) Loosen the clothing.

(*b*) Lay the patient on his back, inclined towards injured side.

(*c*) Give ice to suck, and apply a piece of ice locally over the painful part of the chest.

(*d*) Keep perfectly quiet.

(*e*) Give no stimulants.

(*f*) Apply no bandages, as the pressure of a bandage would be likely to press the displaced end of the broken rib further into the lung.

5. *Fracture of Breast-Bone.*—This is a very rare injury. Pending the arrival of the doctor, all that can be done is to put the patient in an easy position and loosen the clothing.

6. *Fracture of the Collar-Bone.*—

Special Signs.—The arm of the injured side is helpless and the patient droops the shoulder and supports the arm at the elbow with the hand of the sound side.

Treatment.—(1) Remove the patient's coat.

(2) Place a pad about the size of a *small* clenched fist in the armpit.

(3) Bend the elbow and support the limb against the chest.

(4) Apply a "St. John Sling" as follows:—

(*a*) Lay an unfolded triangular bandage across the chest over the injured limb with one end on the uninjured shoulder and the point below the elbow on the injured side.

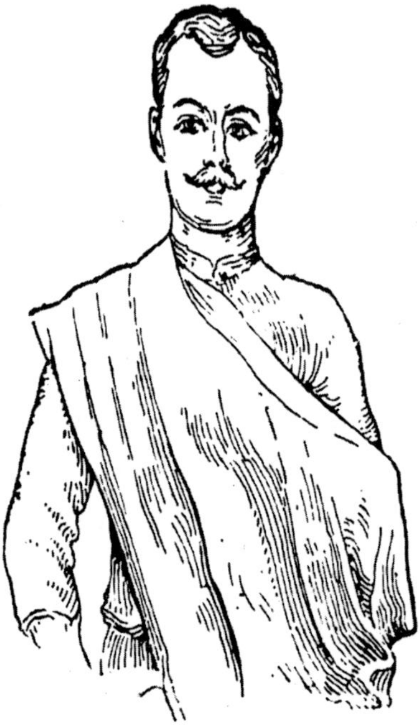

FIG. 23.

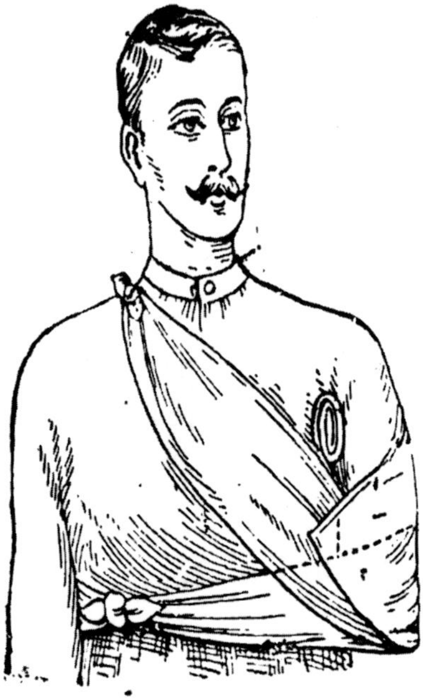

FIG. 24.

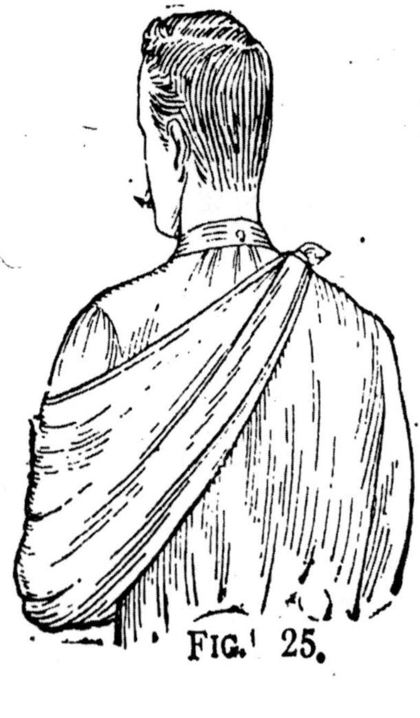

FIG. 25.

FIGS. 23, 24 AND 25. THREE STAGES OF ST. JOHN SLING IN TREATMENT OF FRACTURE OF COLLAR-BONE. (BODY BANDAGE OMITTED TO SHOW DETAILS OF SLING.)

(*b*) Carry the lower end of the bandage under the injured limb, over the back, and tie it off loosely on the top of the sound shoulder.

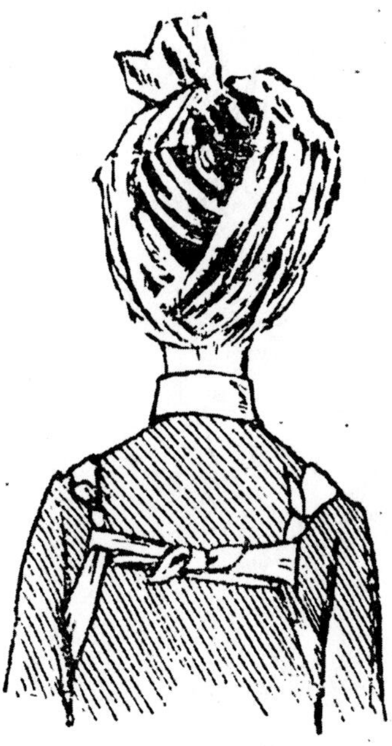

FIG. 26—BANDAGE FOR FRACTURE OF BOTH CLAVICLES.

(*c*) Fold the point forwards over the elbow of the injured limb, and pin.

(*d*) Secure a broad fold bandage round the body just above and over the elbow of the injured side.

(*e*) Tighten the sling so as to support and raise the elbow.

When both collar-bones are broken, four narrow-fold bandages or strips of puggaree are required. One is passed beneath each armpit and made to form a ring round each shoulder; under either ring *behind* the third narrow-fold bandage is slipped, and the ends are pulled tightly and tied in the middle of the back. When both shoulders are secured in position the elbows are bent, the hands crossed over the chest, and the fourth narrow-fold bandage passed round the limbs and body just above the elbows, and tied off in front (Fig. 26.)

7. *Fracture of the Shoulder-Blade.*—This fracture is very rare.

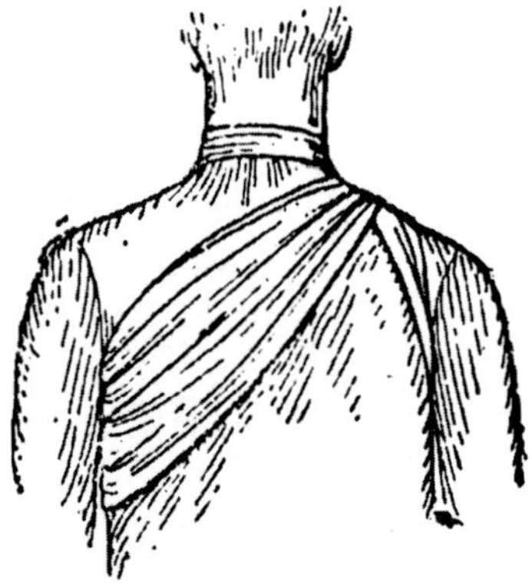

FIG. 27.

BANDAGE FOR FRACTURED SHOULDER-BLADE.

Treatment.—Apply a broad bandage passing it from the armpit of the injured side over the sound shoulder and knot off in the sound armpit. Support the arm on the injured side by means of a "St. John" or great arm sling.

8. *Fracture of the Upper Arm.*—The bone may be broken :—

1. Near the shoulder.
2. About the middle.
3. Near the elbow.

(*a*) *Fracture near Shoulder Joint* :—

1. Apply a broad bandage with its centre on the upper and outer part of the injured arm. Cross the ends in the armpit of the opposite side and tie them off on the top of the sound shoulder

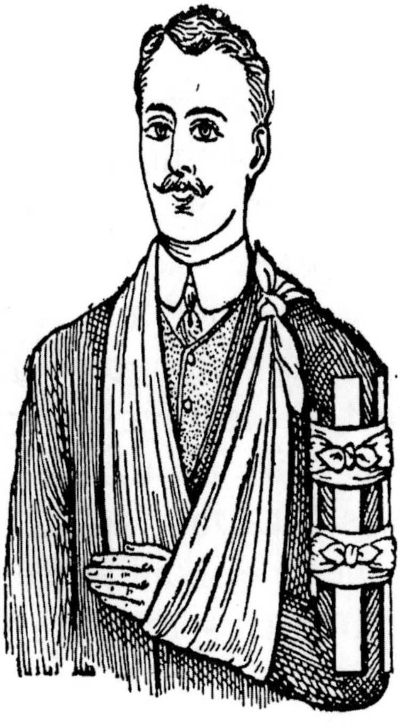

FIG. 28.

TREATMENT OF FRACTURE OF UPPER ARM ABOUT THE MIDDLE.

2. Support the forearm with a small arm sling.

(b) *Fracture about the middle :—*

The forearm is bent at a right angle to the upper arm. Apply four splints extemporised from any handy material, one on each side of, one in front of, and the fourth behind, the upper arm. They should reach from the shoulder to the elbow, except one on the inner side, which must not quite reach to the bend of the elbow. If only two pieces of wood are available, apply them on the inner and outer sides of the arm, as these are the most important places to support. Two pairs of Indian shoes can readily be utilised as four splints. The under surface of the sole should face the skin. When the improvised splints are applied adjust a small arm sling.

If this fracture occurs when travelling and it may be some marches before a doctor's help can be obtained, put up the fracture with the internal angular splint as described for fracture of the elbow.

(c) *Fracture near the Elbow* :—

(1) *If the accident occurs indoors.*—Send immediately for a doctor and pending his arrival place the arm on a pillow and ease the pain by means of ice or cold water dressings.

ANGULAR SPLINT.

(2) *If the accident occurs out of doors.*— Apply an internal angular splint made as follows :—

(*a*) Take two pieces of wood or two bundles of twigs.—One long enough to extend from the armpit to the elbow, and the other long enough to reach from the elbow to the fingers. Tie them together forming the letter " L " and pad well (FIG. 29).

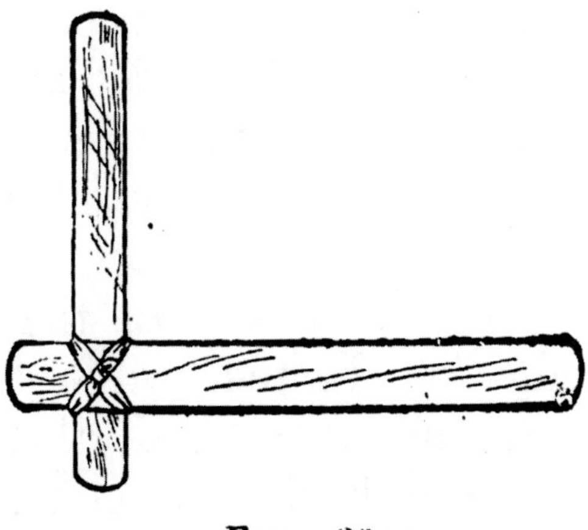

FIG. 29.

(*b*) Bend the elbow into a comfortable position across the chest and apply the apparatus to the inner side of the arm with three or four narrow bandages.

(*c*) Apply a large arm sling.

Remove the splint and treat as under (1) when the patient reaches home.

9. *Fracture of one or both bones of the Forearm.*—When the injury occurs well above the wrist, it is readily recognised. Fractures at or near the wrist are often mistaken for sprains.

Treatment.—(1) Bend the elbow at a right angle. (2) Place the hand with the palm inwards and the thumb upwards. (3) Get someone to hold it in this position. (4) Apply two splints, well padded and slightly broader than the forearm, one splint reaching from the inner side of the elbow to the finger tips, the other extending from the outer side of the elbow to the back of the hand. (5) Fasten with a narrow bandage at the upper end, then at the lower end, and lastly, on either side of the fracture. (6) Adjust a large arm-sling.

It is important in all fractures of the forearm bones that the thumb should be directed upwards and the hand placed with the palm directed to the chest. If the limb is placed so that the palm faces downward the broken ends of the bones overlap and may become welded together in a wrong position and the arm permanently crippled.

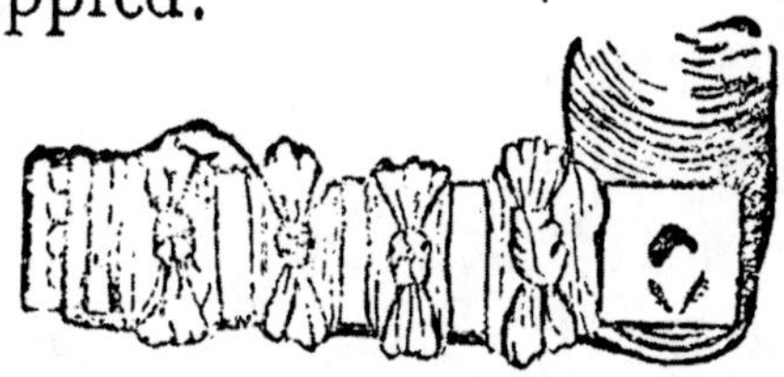

FIG. 30.—TREATMENT OF FRACTURE OF FOREARM.

10. *Crushed Hand—Treatment.*—(1) Lay the whole palm on a broad splint extending from the tips of the fingers to the middle of the forearm. (2) Secure the splint with a narrow bandage applied in the form of a figure of 8. This ensures absolute rest to the fractured finger,

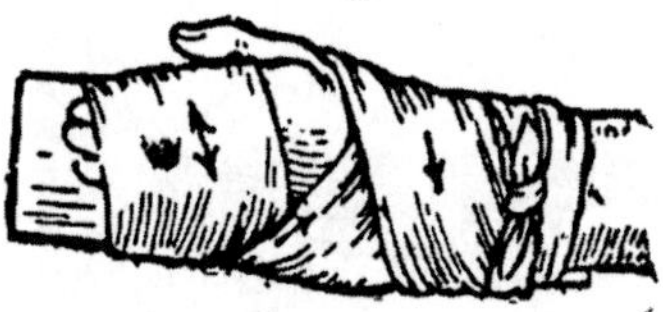

FIG. 31.
TREATMENT OF CRUSHED HAND.

and utilises the adjacent fingers as side splints.

11. *Fracture of the Thigh Bone.*—The bone may be broken at its neck or anywhere in its shaft. The former variety is not uncommon amongst old people and is often the result of quite a slight accident such as tripping or missing a step. The *special signs* are :—

1. The heel cannot be raised from the ground.
2. The foot usually lies on its outer side.

Treatment.—(1) Bring the foot of the injured side into line with the sound side by *gently* and steadily pulling upon it. (2) When it appears to be in position, give it to a helper to keep it steady until splints have

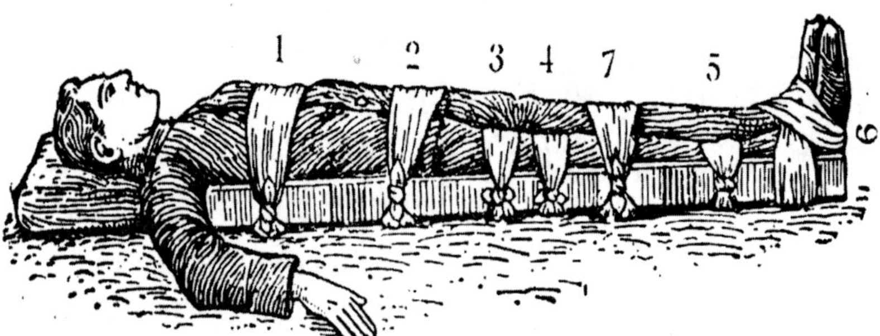

FIG. 32.

SPLINT FOR FRACTURE OF THIGH BONE.

been applied ; or tie the feet together at the ankles.

(*b*) Apply a well-padded lathi or long piece of wood on the outer side of the injured limb, long enough to reach from the armpit to below the foot.

(*c*) Apply a second splint, also well-padded, on the inside of the thigh reaching from the fork to the knee.

(*d*) Secure the splints in position by three broad and four narrow-fold bandages as follows :—No. 1 round the chest just below the armpits, No. 2 round the pelvis. These are the first two broad-fold bandages. Nos. 3, 4, and 5 are narrow-fold bandages. Nos. 3 and 4 round the thigh above and below the fracture, so as to enclose the thigh and both splints. No. 5 round the leg enclosing the long splint. No. 6 secures the ankle to the lower end of the long splint. No. 7 is the third broad-fold bandage. It passes round both knees and secures the injured limb to its fellow. In the case of a woman, the bandages round the thigh and leg should be passed round both limbs, *outside the clothing*, so as to avoid exposure.

12. *Fracture of the Knee Cap.*

Treatment.—(1) Place the patient in a half sitting position so as to relax the muscles of the thigh. (2) Raise the heel by resting it on a box of wood, the sound foot or a folded coat. (3) Apply a back splint broader than the limb at the knee from the hip to the heel. (4) Place a narrow-fold bandage above the broken bone, cross behind the splint, and then tie off in front below the knee. (5) Apply

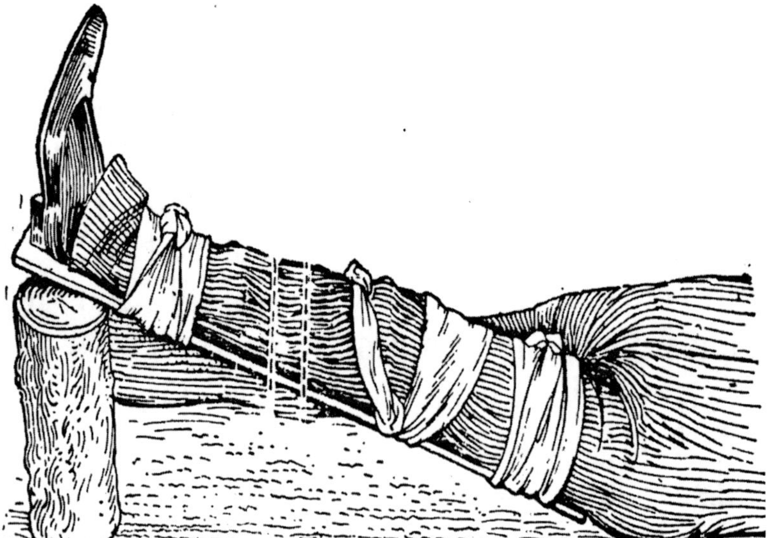

FIG. 33.

TREATMENT OF FRACTURED KNEE CAP.

second bandage in a reverse fashion commencing below the knee, crossing behind and tying off just above the broken bone. Four notches on the edges of the splint where the bandages cross will keep them from slipping.

(6) Secure the splint by one bandage to the thigh and by a second to the foot. (7) Support the foot at a higher level than the rest of the body. (8) Apply ice or cold water dressing to the knee.

13. *Fracture of one or both Bones of the Leg.*—The best method of dealing with this condition is the Edinburgh splint-box

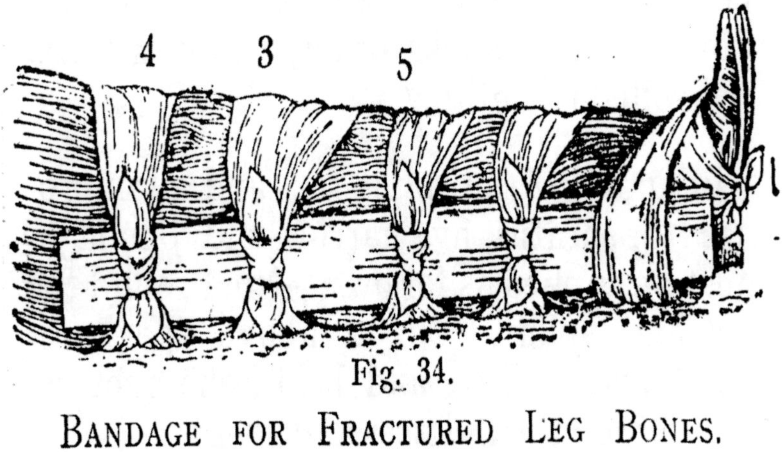

Fig. 34.

BANDAGE FOR FRACTURED LEG BONES.

which is readily improvised as follows:—Two pieces of thin smooth board, wider than the depth of the limb, and reaching from above the knee to below the foot are obtained. An ordinary puggaree or towel is folded to the length of the boards which are rolled up in each end of the towel until a box without ends is formed, which fits the sound leg.

The broken leg is held in proper position and the splint applied. Two small pieces of puggaree or other materials are folded and placed over the front of the leg.

Failing the above simple apparatus, two side splints to reach from above the knee to below the foot must be improvised from sticks or any other material well rolled in clothing.

In applying the splint-box and all improvised apparatus, five narrow-fold bandages must be applied as follows:—No. 1 round the foot and splint. No. 2 above the knee. Nos. 3 and 4 above and below the fracture. No. 5 round both knees and splint.

14. *Fracture or Crushed Bones of the Foot.*—Usually caused by a heavy weight falling on the foot. Readily recognised by pain, swelling and inability to use the foot.

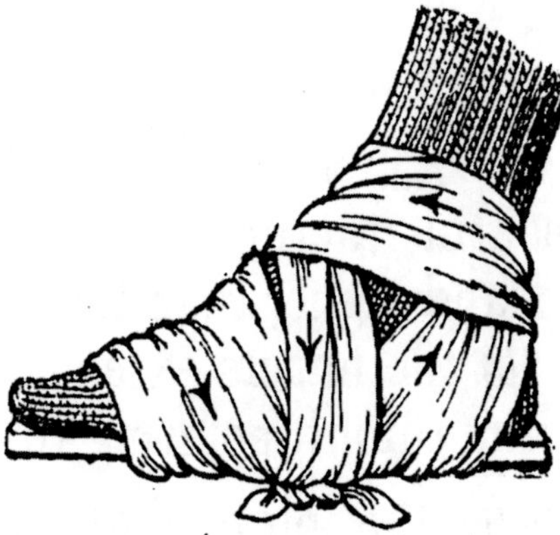

FIG. 35.

TREATMENT OF CRUSHED FOOT.

Treatment :—

(1) Rip up back seam of boot and cut off sock.

(2) Apply a well-padded piece of wood to foot.

(3) Apply a figure of eight bandage, as shown by arrows in Fig. 35.

(4) Elevate the foot.

The First-Aider must remember always:—

(1) To pad his splints.

(2) To apply his bandages and tie them off *over* his splint.

(3) In leg fractures to set the foot at right angles to the leg.

(4) In arm fractures to (*a*) place the hand higher than the elbow with (*b*) the fingers extended and (*c*) the thumb pointing to the chin.

(5) To fix the joints above and below the fracture with his splint and not to apply a splint over a wound.

CHAPTER VI.

Dislocations, Sprains and Strains.

Dislocations.—When, as the result of an injury the ligaments of a joint are torn, the bones usually slip out of place and what is known as a *dislocation* occurs. Some joints are much more liable to dislocation than others; "ball-and-socket" joints on account of their extensive range of movement are more frequently dislocated than "hinge-joints," for instance, dislocation of the shoulder-joint is a common injury compared with dislocation of the elbow-joint.

The following are the signs and symptoms of dislocation :—

1. Pain in and around the joint. This is usually of a sickening character.

2. Change in the shape of the joint.

3. Swelling round the joint.

4. Fixity of the joint. All the usual movements are impossible.

5. Alteration in the length of the limb, *i.e.*, lengthening or shortening.

6. Numbness and uselessness of the limb.

Treatment :—

(*a*) *Out of doors.*—Support the limb in a comfortable position.

(*b*) *Indoors.*—(1) Send for Surgeon. (2) Remove clothing and put the patient to bed. (3) Place the limb on pillow and apply ice or cold water dressing. (4) If cold fails to give relief, apply hot fomentations. (5) Avoid shock by keeping the patient warm.

Sprains.—A sprain is an injury of a joint involving tearing of the ligaments.

Strains.—A strain is merely the *over-stretching* of a muscle or tendon.

The signs of sprain are familiar, *viz.* :—

1. Pain.
2. Inability to move the joint, muscle or tendon.
3. Swelling and discolouration.

Sprained ankle is the commonest sprain. The treatment is as follows :—

(*a*) *Out of doors.*—(1) Don't remove boot. (2) Apply a tight bandage over the boot beginning at the sole, crossing in front of the ankle and passing several times round the ankle. (3) Wet the bandage after application as this tightens it.

(*b*) *Indoors.*—(1) Remove boot as in crushed foot. (2) Place in a comfortable position. (3) Apply cold water bandages. If these fail to give relief, use hot formentations.

Strains are treated by resting the limb in a comfortable position or going to bed. Hot applications usually give most relief.

CHAPTER VII.

THE HEART AND BLOOD VESSELS.

The heart is the central pump by which the circulation is carried on. It is envelop-ed in a completely closed bag of membrane consisting of two layers, the outer of which is attached to surrounding structures. The heart is conical in shape, about the size of the closed fist, and consists of a hollow in-voluntary muscle, containing four chambers, two on each side. The upper chambers are known as the right and left *auricles* and the lower as the right and left *ventricles.* There is no communication be-tween the chambers of the right and those of the left side. The ventricles are supplied with valves at their inlet and outlet openings, each inlet thus allowing the blood to flow from the auricle into the ventricle below it, but not back again, and each outlet allowing it to flow on into an outlet artery, but permitting no reflux.

The Circulation of the Blood.—Starting from the left ventricle, the blood is propelled

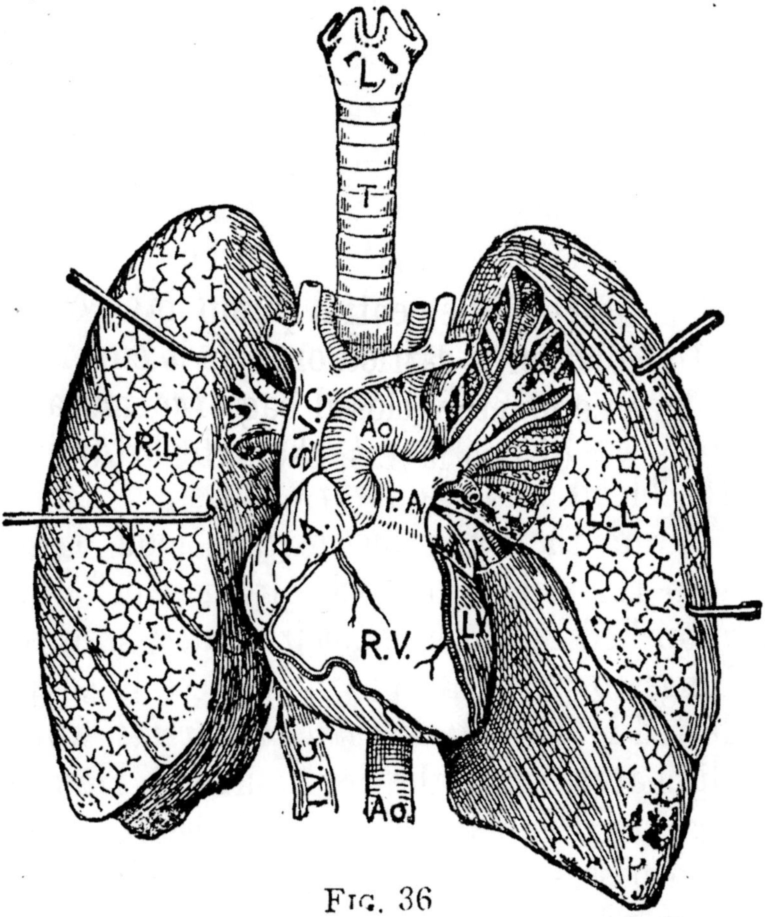

FIG. 36

L. Larynx (voice box) ; T. Trachea (wind-pipe); R. L. Right Lung ; L. L. Left Lung (the lungs are drawn back to expose the heart and blood vessels); **R. A.** Right Auricle ; L. A. Left Auricle ; R. V. Right Ventricle ; L. V. Left Ventricle ; **P.** A. Pulmonary Artery ; Ao, Aorta ; S. V. C. Superior vena cava (the large vein carrying blood from the upper part of the body to the heart) ; I. V. C. Inferior vena cava (the large vein carrying blood from the lower part of the body to the heart). The four pulmonary veins cannot be shown in the Diagram.

into a large artery called the *Aorta* which divides into several branches, some carrying the blood to the upper, and one large one to the lower part of the body. From the arteries the blood flows into the capillaries and thence into the veins which finally discharge into two main veins *the Superior and Inferior Vena Cava,* which conduct the blood into the right auricle.

From the right auricle the blood passes into the right ventricle, from which it is propelled by the *Pulmonary Artery* into the lungs to be purified: from these it is collected into the four *pulmonary veins* which discharge into the left auricle. Here it reaches the left side of the heart again, and passes into the left ventricle, the point from which we started. See Fig. 36 which illustrates all these structures.

A complete circulation of the blood takes place in 20 to 30 heart beats (Cleland). The heart beats on the average 75 times a minute in adults. In infants the rate is 120 a minute.

The Blood Vessels.—The tubes that carry the blood are of three kinds :—(1) Arteries,

(2) capillaries, and (3) veins.

(1) *The Arteries.*—The arteries are elastic tubes, and when the heart propels the arterial blood through them, they yield and expand, thus giving rise to the movement of the arteries, known as the pulse. It is usual to feel the pulse at the wrist, but the movement can be felt and counted in any position where an artery passes over a bone. From the large arteries the blood is propelled into the smaller, until it reaches—

(2) *The Capillaries.*—These are minute vessels in which the interchange of the products of waste and repair takes place, and the pure arterial blood becomes converted into the impure venous blood. From the capillaries the blood flows into—

(3) *The Veins.*—The veins gradually increasing in size towards the heart. They are not elastic like the arteries and are supplied with structures called valves which open towards the heart and permit of blood flowing only in that direction. The valves are composed of two pouches, which, when filled with blood, belly out, join, and prevent any further return of blood towards

the capillaries. When these valves become inefficient the vein becomes changed in character and shape and becomes what is called a varicose vein. The veins usually accompany the arteries and bear the same name. In some parts of the body an artery is accompanied by two veins.

The General Course of the Arteries.—The *Aorta* or main artery from the left ventricle of the heart and arching backwards lies chiefly along the front of the spine, giving out branches to all parts of the body.

These branches pass upwards, outwards and downwards, and it should be remembered that as a river gets different names in various parts of its course, so the arteries are really continuous streams of blood getting special names from the parts they traverse.

(1) *Upwards* pass the two *Carotid* arteries, supplying the head. The branch of the carotid in the region of the temple is called the *temporal* artery and the branch on the face the *facial* artery.

Outwards passes the great artery supplying the upper limb acquiring special names from the adjacent bones, or the regions through which it passes. Thus it is called the *Subclavian*, as it passes underneath the collarbone. A little further on, the same vessel passes through the armpit, under the name of the *Axillary* artery. We next find it lying in the arm, under the name of the *Brachial* artery. At the elbow it forks into two branches, *Radial* and *Ulnar*, deriving their names from the bones of the forearm. In the palm of the hand the continuation of the outer of these forms an arch called the *Palmer* arch, from which branches are given off to the fingers.

Downwards, the main artery terminates in arteries which pass to the flanks, called the *Right and Left Common Iliac* arteries. Each of these divide into two, *viz.*, the *Internal Iliac* artery which supplies blood to the bladder, bowel and other contents of the pelvis and the *External Iliac* which is continued down the front of the thigh as the *Femoral* artery, deriving its name from the femur or thigh bone. Dipping through the thigh, it makes its appearance again behind the knee as the artery of the ham called the *Popliteal* artery. In this position it forks, its branches distributing themselves to the back and front of the leg under the names of *Anterior and Posterior Tibial* arteries and are continued down to the foot, similarly to the arteries of the arm and hand.

The First Aid student must remember that the *Femoral* artery crosses the brim of the pelvis at a point found by taking the centre of a line drawn from the prominent point of the haunch bone to a position immediately about the private parts.

In the groin its position is indicated by a line drawn from the centre of the groin to the back of the inner side of the knee.

CHAPTER VIII.

HÆMORRHAGE.

Varieties.—There are three varieties of hæmorrhage, *viz.*—(1) Arterial, (2) Venous, and (3) Capillary. It is important to distinguish between these, as the methods for arresting bleeding are different in each variety.

(1) *Arterial Hæmorrhage.*—When an artery is wounded, the blood is recognised by the following characteristics:—(*a*) It is bright red, (*b*) it escapes from the wounded vessel in spurts or jets corresponding to the beats of the heart, (*c*) it issues from the end of the vessel next the heart.

(2) *Venous Hæmorrhage.*—In bleeding from a vein the blood is (*a*) dark purple in colour, (*b*) it flows from the wound in a continuous stream, (*c*) it issues from the end further from the heart except in wounds of varicose veins when it escapes from both sides.

(3) *Capillary Hæmorrhage.*—In this variety the blood is bright red, and oozes

from all parts of the wound, trickling by gravitation down to the deeper parts.

The General Means of Arresting Hæmorrhage.

1. *Position.*—The bleeding part must be kept in an elevated position, as blood finds greater difficulty in flowing upwards. If an arm is wounded, it must be supported in a sling; if a leg, the patient must be made to lie down with the limb raised on a pillow.

2. *Cold.*—The action of cold in the form of ice or iced water in arresting bleeding is due to a stimulating effect on the ends of the bleeding vessels which contract and prevent the escape of blood.

3. *Pressure.*—This is effected by the fingers, by pads and bandages, and other appliances, such as tourniquets. Its object is to favour contraction of the cut ends of the bleeding vessels and promote clot.

For each artery there is a special point at which pressure should be applied when the artery is wounded. This place is called the *pressure point* and is indicated in the frontispiece and described in the Table on p. 78 (*a*).

The Treatment of Arterial Hæmorrhage.

In the treatment of this variety of hæmorrhage, general means 1 and 2 may be ignored, and we must rely on pressure which may be exercised by :—

(*a*) The fingers and thumb.
(*b*) Pad and bandage.
(*c*) The graduated compress.
(*d*) Forcible bending of the joints.
(*e*) Tourniquets, which are of three varieties, *viz.*:—

(1) The St. John Tourniquet.
(2) Screw.
(3) Improvised.

(*a*) *Digital pressure or pressure with the fingers or thumb.*—So long as we can place a finger on the mouth of a bleeding artery, we need have no fear of hæmorrhage. The finger and thumb, therefore, are the most efficient and handy First Aid tools we possess.

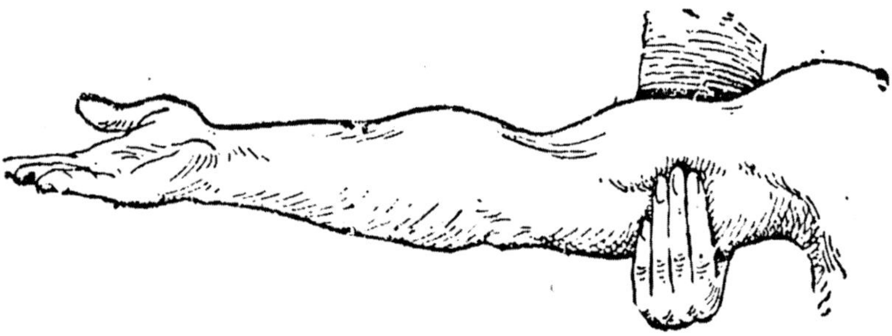

FIG. 37.

DIGITAL COMPRESSION OF THE BRACHIAL ARTERY.

Finger pressure may be made either directly over the bleeding artery, or in some convenient part of its course, where, from its nearness to the surface and its proximity to a bone, it can be effectually pressed against the latter.

(*b*) *Pad and Bandage.*—Pads may be extemporised from handkerchiefs, neckties, or pieces of puggaree rolled up tightly. They may readily be made firmer by enclosing in them stones, corks, coins, or pieces of wood.

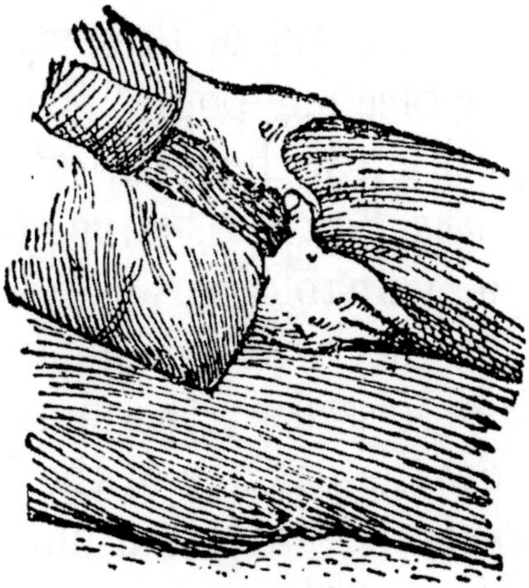

Fig. 38.

DIGITAL COMPRESSION OF THE FEMORAL ARTERY.

The pad should be secured by a narrow-fold bandage applied so as to press it firmly against the bleeding point.

(*c*) *The Graduated Compress.*—In some parts of the body, especially the palm of the hand, what is called a *graduated compress* is more effective than a simple pad. It is made by cutting a number of pads of *clean* lint or linen of similar shape but gradually diminishing in size; the smallest being about as big as a four-anna piece. The pads are applied one on top of the other so as to form a little pyramid of dressings with its apex over the bleeding point. The compress is kept in position with a strip of puggaree.

(*d*) *Pad and Forced Bending of the Joint.* —This is a valuable means of arresting hæmorrhage, the artery being so sharply bent and compressed by the muscles that it will not allow the passage of the blood.

(*e*) *Tourniquets.*—A tourniquet is an apparatus for applying and maintaining pressure over an artery.

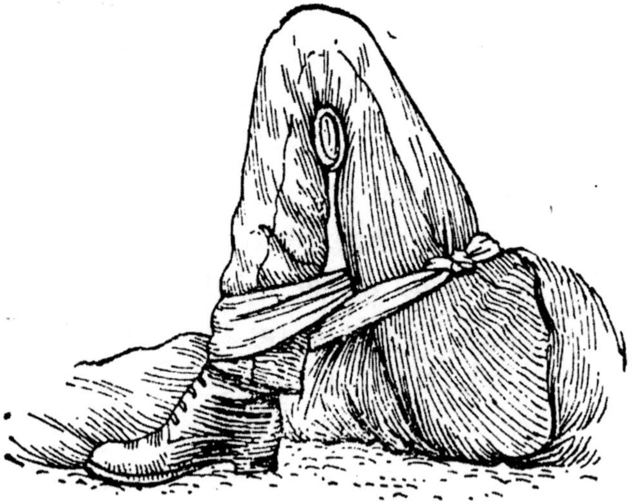

FIG. 39.

PAD IN HAM AND FLEXION FOR WOUND OF LEG.

There are three chief types :—

(1) *The St. John Tourniquet.*—This consists of a pad, strap, buckle, "D" and string running in a piece of cane. It is applied as follows :—

1. Place the rounded side of the pad on the pressure point.

2. Pass strap round the limb and buckle it.

3. After noting that the pad is in the correct position apply sufficient pressure by means of the twisting apparatus to arrest hæmorrhage. The twisting apparatus should be kept as near the centre of the pad as possible. Should moderate pressure fail to arrest hæmorrhage it may be assumed that the pad is incorrectly placed.

4. Pass the appropriate end of the string, which runs freely within the cane, through the "D" attached to the buckle and tie it. To ensure ease in relaxing pressure the hitch or knot securing the string should be finished with a loop.

5. If medical assistance is not available within half an hour, relax pressure for a few moments; if hæmorrhage occurs again

tighten the tourniquet.

This apparatus is used in the Royal Navy and can be obtained for twelve annas from the Indian Headquarters of the S. J. Ambulance Association.

2. *The Screw Tourniquet.*—This consists of a strap and buckle to surround the limb, a pad to press on the artery and a screw arrangement to tighten the strap and increase the pressure on the artery.

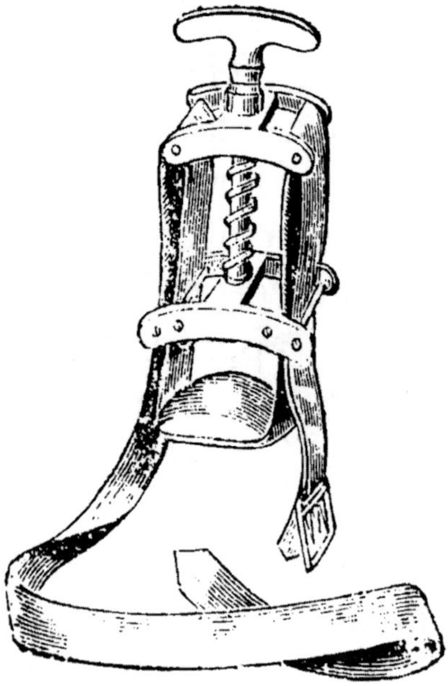

FIG. 40.—THE SCREW TOURNIQUET.

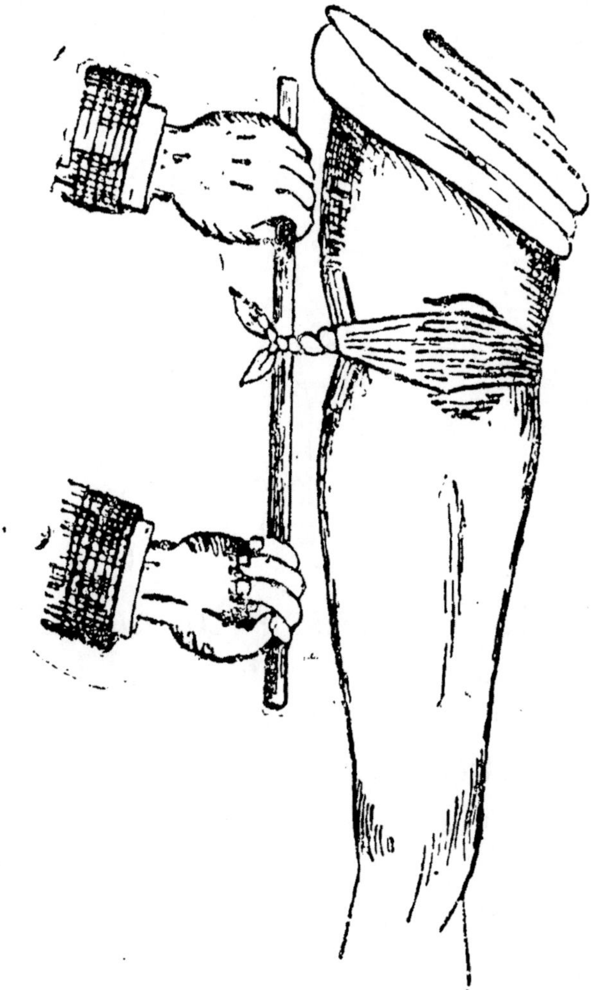

FIG. 41.—IMPROVISED TOURNIQUET FOR COMPRESSION OF WOUNDS OF THE FEMORAL ARTERY.

3. *The Improvised Tourniquet.*—This is the most useful variety for First Aid purposes.

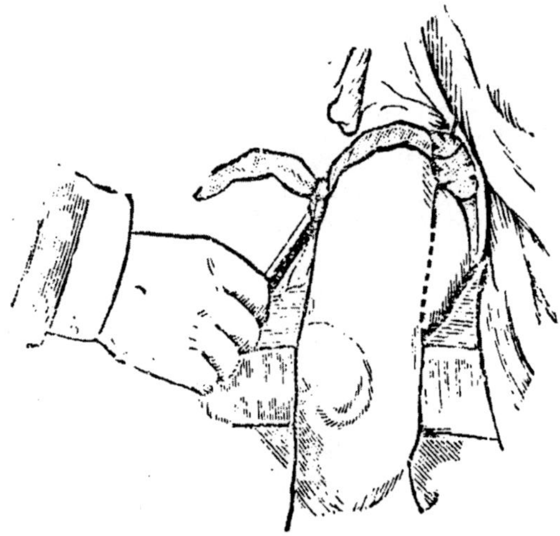

FIG. 42—IMPROVISED TOURNIQUET.

It consists essentially of a pad to place over the artery, a narrow bandage and a piece of stick. An ordinary pad and bandage may be converted into a tourniquet by introducing a stout pencil into the knot and twisting it until sufficient pressure is exerted to stop the bleeding. Where a suitable pad is not available, a knot may be tied on a narrow bandage and applied over the artery. It is very important that the pressure should be exactly over the artery, otherwise the bleeding will continue.

The arrest of Bleeding in the various parts of the Body.

	Part wounded.	The pressure-point.	The direction of pressure.	The method of applying pressure.	The mode of applying bandage.
1.	Front or top of the head.	Just in front of the lappet guarding the opening of the ear.	Directly against the bone.	(i) By finger. (ii) A pad placed on the artery by means of a triangular bandage.	Narrow-fold bandage twisted so as to maintain firm pressure.
2.	The back of the head.	Two fingers' breadth behind the back of the ear.	Ditto.	Ditto.	Centre of narrow-fold bandage on pad, cross on forehead and knot off on pad.
3.	The neck ..	The hollow just on outer side of Adam's apple.	Backwards and inwards against the backbone. Pressure on the wind-pipe must be carefully avoided.	With the finger, to be maintained by relays of capable assistants. Bend the head forward upon the chest and fix it in this position by means of bandages and pillows.	Maintain pressure yourself or get a helper to do so, till doctor arrives. Do not apply a bandage.
4.	The armpit ..	The hollow just above and behind the centre of the collar-bone.	Downwards and backwards against the upper surface of first rib.	With the thumbs at first, then with the handle of a door-key *padded*.	Place pad in armpit and keep in position with a narrow bandage crossed over the shoulder and knotted off under opposite armpit. Apply large arm sling.
5.	The arm above the elbow.	The hollow just below the biceps muscle.	Outwards and backwards against the arm bone.	(i) Stand behind patient. (ii) Grasp arm, pressing tips of fingers along inner side of biceps muscle. (iii) Rotate arm outwards and backwards.	Place a firm pad over the line of the brachial artery and keep in position with narrow bandage. Place forearm in a large sling.
6.	The forearm ..	At the bend of the elbow.	Downwards and backwards against the bone.	Apply pad made from folded handkerchief to bend of elbow. Flex the forearm firmly on the arm.	Pass a narrow bandage or belt round forearm close to wrists and carry ends just below the armpit. Bring ends forward again crossing between forearm and arm and tie off over wrists.
7.	The palm of hand.	Half an inch above the wrist on each side.	Elevate the arm and press directly backwards against the wrist bones.	With the fingers at first, afterwards with pad, or graduated compress.	Place a rolled-up handkerchief in the palm, bend the fingers over it and apply bandage firmly. If bleeding continues, proceed as for bleeding from forearm.
8.	The thigh (high up).	Just below the centre of the fold of groin.	Bend the knee and turn the thigh outwards and then press outwards towards the thigh bone.	With both thumbs, one upon the other; keep up pressure by relays of trained helpers.	A bandage should not be applied, but pressure should be maintained either by yourself or a trained helper till doctor arrives.
9.	The ham ..	Four fingers' breadth below the fold of the groin.	Do.	With tourniquet.	Narrow bandage as in Fig. 42.
10.	The leg ..	In the centre of the ham.	Directly backwards against the bone as much as possible.	With both thumbs, one upon the other, then use a tourniquet. Pad as large as a golf ball behind the knee. Bend the knee until the heel almost touches the hip.	Carry round leg just above ankle and tie round thigh as close to groin as possible (see page 74.)
11.	The foot ..	(i) In the hollow behind the prominence of inner ankle. (ii) Over the centre of the ankle in front.	Raise legs, press forwards and outwards against the bone for (i), and directly backwards against the bone for (ii).	Apply a pad on each pressure-point and bandage in this position.	Apply centre of narrow bandage to sole of foot, cross over the pads, carry round the ankle and tie off over pads.

The pupil should commit the following rules for arresting arterial hæmorrhage to memory :—

1. Apply pressure with the finger or thumb whilst a pad is being prepared.
2. Apply pad over the bleeding point and bandage firmly.
3. If this procedure fails, try pad and forcible bending of joint above the wound.
4. If this fails apply pressure at the pressure point by means of the fingers or a St. John, or improvised, tourniquet.

The table on page 78(*a*) indicates the treatment for arterial bleeding in any part of the body,

THE ARREST OF VENOUS HÆMORRHAGE.

1. *Normal Veins.*—This is never so serious as arterial hæmorrhage and can usually be arrested by—

1. Applying the thumb to the bleeding point.
2. A pad and bandage.

3. In the event of oozing taking place after the application of the pad and bandage, do not remove it, but apply a narrow bandage firmly round the limb on the side furthest from the heart.

2. *Varicose Veins* :—These are veins in the leg which from one of many causes become increased in length and dilated. Owing to increase in length the veins become twisted and curved in order to fit into their allotted space. The skin over these vessels, because of the bad circulation, may ulcerate and the covering over the vein become so thin that a slight injury may burst open the vein leading to very serious hæmorrhage as the valves having disappeared the blood comes from both sides of the vein.

The treatment of the serious emergency of hæmorrhage from a varicose vein is as follows :—

1. Lay the patient down.
2. Raise the leg.
3. Remove the clothing.
4. Apply pressure with the thumb.

5. Dress with a pad and bandage.
6. Should oozing continue after the application of the pad, apply a narrow-fold bandage firmly round the limb *both above and below* the bleeding point.

The Treatment of Capillary Hæmorrhage.

1. If practicable, raise the bleeding part.
2. Apply pressure either by means of a perfectly *clean* finger, or a *clean* piece of linen rag or lint.
3. Keep the dressing in position with a narrow bandage.

Internal Hæmorrhage.

This is a very serious condition and may be either arterial, venous or capillary.

It may be from the lungs when the blood is scarlet and frothy and coughed up, or from the stomach when it is dark in colour, and vomited, or from the other organs when it is not seen.

The signs are :—

1. Fainting and giddiness.
2. The breathing becomes shallow and hurried.
3. The patient yawns and sighs.
4. The pulse becomes weak.
5. The lips become ashy grey.
6. Cold clammy sweat breaks out.
7. The patient complains of being suffocated, gasps for air, and may become unconscious.

Treatment :—

1. Send for a doctor.
2. Keep the patient quiet and lying down.
3. Loosen anything tight about the neck or body.
4. Give small pieces of ice to suck.
5. Do not give stimulants.
6. If the patient is on a charpoy, raise the foot of it.
7. Keep him absolutely quiet and avoid all conversation with him.
8. Gently restrain him should he become restless.

9. Do everything to allay anxiety should he become worried about his condition.

Bleeding from the Nose.

Treatment :—

1. Seat the patient in a chair in the open or before an open window, with the head slightly thrown back.
2. Raise the hands above the head and give them to an assistant to hold.
3. Undo all tight clothing around the neck and chest.
4. Apply a cold sponge or a piece of ice over the nose and also at the back of the neck.
5. Instruct the patient to keep his mouth open, so as to avoid breathing through the nose.
6. Place the feet in hot water.

CHAPTER IX.

Wounds, Bites and Stings.

Wounds are injuries of the body with more or less division of the skin.

Varieties of Wounds.—There are five kinds of wounds, each having special characters of its own, and therefore requiring different kinds of treatment :—

1. Incised.
2. Lacerated.
3. Contused.
4. Punctured.
5. Gunshot.

Any of these five varieties may, by the entrance of microbes, become poisoned.

The general treatment of all kinds is :—

1. To arrest the bleeding.
2. To cleanse the wound.
3. To protect the wound from becoming poisoned.
4. If possible, to keep the wounded parts at rest by the application of splints or slings.
5. To treat constitutional symptoms, if present, such as shock or syncope.

The most important of these points to remember is to avoid *touching* any wound *with dirty hands,* as doing so will poison it, and the smallest poisoned wound is more serious than the largest clean cut. Tincture of Iodine is of the greatest value in preventing all wounds from becoming poisoned. In India it should be kept in every household and workshop and all cuts, and even scratches, painted with it.

1. *Incised Wounds.*—These are wounds inflicted with sharp instruments. The amount of bleeding varies with the depth of the wound and the part injured.

Treatment.—Arrest the bleeding and apply Tincture of Iodine and clean lint. If these are not available, then apply a piece of clean paper such as the inside of an envelope and keep it on with a strip of puggaree or a handkerchief folded as a triangular bandage.

2. *Lacerated Wounds.*—When the skin and parts beneath are torn by machinery or other cause, and the surface of the wound is jagged or ragged, this condition is described as a lacerated wound.

Treatment.—Apply Tincture of Iodine, envelop the whole wound in some clean linen and prepare for hæmorrhage which may come on after the person has recovered from the shock of the injury.

3. *Contused Wounds.*—These are usually due to a blow with a club, *lathi* or other blunt weapon. Wounds with a club on the scalp may appear clean cut and look like incised wounds.

Treatment.—The treatment is the same as for lacerated wounds.

4. *Punctured Wounds.*—A stab with any sharp instrument produces a punctured wound.

Bleeding may be slight, but shock severe.

Treatment.—Remove the weapon if present, apply Tincture of Iodine and cover the wound up.

5. *Gunshot Wounds.*—The injuries produced by all varieties of firearms are called gunshot wounds.

(*a*) *Shot Wounds.*—When a person is peppered with shot from a sporting gun, if the wound is not properly cleansed, the formation of matter may follow; and an abscess or general blood poisoning supervene.

Treatment.—The best treatment is to paint the wounded part with Tincture of Iodine and then to wrap it up in a towel or *clean* puggaree wrung out of hot water. Pellets easily reached may be extracted, but shot buried in the fleshy parts of the body should be left alone as they cause little inconvenience.

(*b*) *Bullet Wounds.*—As a rule there are two wounds, a small one where the bullet enters, and a larger one where it leaves the body. With the present-day high velocity small bore rifles there is but little difference between the wound of entrance and exit.

The *treatment* is :—

1. Arrest bleeding.
2. Paint with Tincture of Iodine.
3. Cover up quickly.
4. Apply splints as for fracture.
5. Treat the shock which is always present.

Poisoned Wounds.—These are produced from any of the five previous varieties of wounds by the introduction of dirt and microbes.

Treatment.—Wash the wound with carbolic lotion (1 in 40), or Tincture of Iodine, one teaspoonful to half a pint of water, and dress with sterilised lint.

Should any wound and the parts surrounding it become hot, swollen or painful and medical advice is not obtainable, foment it by applying boric lint wrung out of boiling water. Cover the lint with some waterproof material and keep it in position with a strip of bandage.

Abdominal Wounds.

A word or two is required on the subject of Abdominal Wounds in which more or less of the abdominal contents escape through a large wound.

1. Send a written message to a doctor describing the injury at once.

2. Place a clean cloth over the wound and keep it constantly wet with a weak solution of salt and warm water, (strength : a teaspoonful of salt to a pint of water), for if the delicate structures of the bowel become dry they will suffer almost fatal

damage from this cause alone.

3. If the wound of the abdomen is transverse, roll up a coat or small durrie and place it under the knees so as to bend them and thus, by relaxing the muscles of the belly, bring the lips of the abdominal wound together.

4. Treat shock as laid down on page 103.

Bites and Stings.

Stings of Insects.—The sting of a bee, wasp, or hornet may occasion severe symptoms and has actually resulted in death.

The symptoms when severe are those of shock accompanied by vomiting, swelling of the face, hands and feet, and delirium.

Treatment.—Endeavour to extract the sting by squeezing the part stung with the finger and thumb or by pressing the hollow part of the stem of a small key against it, wash the wound with a weak solution of ammonia, whisky or any form of spirits, and rub in permanganate of potash. Tincture of Iodine is one of the best applications to all kinds of stings.

Avert shock by keeping the patient warm, making him lie down and giving stimulants.

SNAKE BITE :—

Treatment :—

The bite of a poisonous snake is recognised by its producing two small bleeding points about one inch apart.

1. Send for medical assistance stating why the doctor is wanted.

2. Meanwhile apply a piece of string or a narrow-fold triangular bandage tightly round the limb or finger between the wound and the heart, to prevent general absorption of the snake poison into the system and another similar construction higher up. It is best to apply this second bandage above the knee in the case of bites of the foot and leg, and above the elbow in bites of the hand and forearm.

3. Administer stimulants to counteract failure of the heart.

4. Allow the wounded part to hang down and bathe it with warm water to encourage bleeding and so wash the poison out of the wound.

5. Make a cross-shaped cut over the points where the fang entered and rub in crystals of permanganate of potash which destroy the snake poison.

6. Perform artificial respiration if the patient becomes unconscious.

Bites of Mad Dogs.—In India a dog-bite must always be regarded as dangerous. In no case should the dog be destroyed. It should be kept tied up under observation for at least ten days. If during that time the dog dies without any apparent cause it will generally be found that it is rabid. Bites on the head, face and neck are especially dangerous.

Treatment :—

1. Apply two constrictions round the limbs as indicated for snake-bite.

2. Wash the wound well with warm water to encourage bleeding.

3. Cauterise with pure carbolic acid or some fluid caustic such as nitric acid. *Do not rely on lunar caustic.*

4. Send the person to the nearest Pasteur Institute within four days in the case

of bites on the head or face or in the case of bites on other parts of the body if the medical authorities think that the dog is mad.

Bites of Centipedes, Tarantulas, Spiders, &c.—Treat these exactly similarly to snake-bite. Permanganate of Potash has power to neutralise the poison of all venomous bites *with the exception of dog-bite.*

Scorpion Sting.—At the end of the tail of the scorpion there is a sting having a small central canal (which communicates with the poison-secreting organ). Through this canal the poison is conveyed to the part stung. The pain produced is sometimes intense and occasionally scorpion sting is fatal in children. The sting is at first like the prick of a sharp needle followed by a sensation as if a number of needles were being inserted ; the pain shoots up the limb, and there is soon some swelling and irritation of the part stung.

The best applications are Scrubb's ammonia on lint, Sal volatile or Solution of ammonia, Eau-de-Cologne, the cut surface of a raw onion or tobacco juice; and afterwards a lotion of spirit (brandy or whisky) and water, or a laudanum fomentation.* If seen early after the sting, sucking the wound often relieves the pain.

Fish-hook in Finger.—When a boy gets a fish-hook in his finger do not attempt to draw it out the way it went in. Cut the dressing off the hook, leaving only the metal, push the barbed point through the skin and the remainder of the hook will readily follow it. Wash the wound well, paint with Tincture of Iodine and dress as an ordinary wound.

---

* See *Indian Home Nursing*, 3rd Edition, page 135.

CHAPTER X.

BRUISES, BURNS AND SCALDS.

Bruises.—These are due to bleeding underneath the skin consequent on the rupture of minute blood-vessels. The injured part is at first reddened by the blow, but quickly becomes purple in hue and afterwards almost black.

The black fades to violet in the third day, to a greenish tint on the fifth to the seventh day, becomes yellow about the eighth or tenth, and gradually fades to the normal colour of the skin on the thirteenth to eighteenth day. A "black-eye" shows all these shades of colouring very well.

The Treatment of Bruises.—This consists in applying cold in some form or other. Tincture of Arnica has a great household reputation in the treatment of bruises. This is due to the fact that it is made from strong spirit which, when mixed with water, produces a compound which rapidly evaporates and thus produces more cold than an ordinary water bandage. Eau de Cologne and water constitute a much pleasanter and equally efficacious application, while methylated spirit and water can be used where economy is an object. Raw meat is believed by school boys to be a sovereign remedy for a black-eye, but the only virtue of raw meat in this relation is that it is cold.

Burns and Scalds.—A burn is produced by flames, hot metals and similar *dry* substances, whereas a scald is produced by boiling water, hot oil, molten metal, tar and similar liquids.

If slight, the effect on the body is to produce simple reddening, but if more severe, blebs or " blisters " are formed.

Treatment :—

1. *To remove the clothing.*—If stuck to the skin, the clothing must be cut all round the burn and left to come off of its own accord. If the foot is scalded, the First Aider must not attempt to remove the boot in the ordinary way, but must undo the lace and cut the back seam of the boot so

that the boot may fall off of its own accord. The stocking must also be cut along the back so as to come off readily.

2. Do not prick the blisters, but cover up the wound with small pieces of lint or linen soaked in salad oil or any other variety of vegetable or animal oil which may be handy. One of the best applications is an emulsion made of equal parts of salad or linseed oil and lime water. When the burnt surface is extensive, use several small pieces of lint instead of one large piece, so that in subsequent dressings the wound may be dressed a small piece at a time; by doing this the shock to the system, which is the great risk of burns, is much less than if the whole burnt surface is exposed at one time.

When the hand or foot is burnt, place it in warm water to which a little bicarbonate of soda has been added, or in weak carbolic lotion (1 in 80) while the oily dressings are being got ready. This greatly eases the pain of the burn. If the face is burnt, cut holes in a piece of lint for the eyes, mouth and nose, smear the lint with vaseline containing half a drachm to the ounce of eucalyptus oil and tie it on with tapes.

3. The severe shock which accompanies every burn of any magnitude must be dealt with by wrapping the person in warm blankets, putting a couple of hot-water bottles in the bed, giving plenty of warm milk, hot clear soup, or hot coffee.

Slight burns of the neck often cause severe symptoms.

What to do when clothing catches fire.—Pick up a rug, tablecloth or blanket and hold it between the person and yourself. (2) Throw the person on the floor so that the flames are uppermost. (3) Roll the burning clothing in a rug or blanket until the fire is quite extinguished.

In the case of Women.—Should your own dress catch fire (1) lie down as fire ascends, (2) wrap yourself round in a durrie, rug or blanket, or, failing that, in the sound part of your dress. (3) On no account rush out of doors as the air will feed the flames.

Scalds of the Throat.—This accident is not infrequent in Europe from children drinking water from the spout of a kettle or teapot full of boiling water.

Treatment.—(1) Apply a piece of flannel or a sponge wrung out of warm water to the front of the throat.

(2) Give the child ice to suck or cold water to sip.

(3) Keep it warm and out of draughts.

The causes of the various kinds of INSENSIBILITY, the means of recognising them, and their special treatment.

	HEAD INJURIES.		FITS.					EFFECTS OF HEAT, SEVERE INJURIES, ALCOHOL AND POISONS.			
	Concussion of Brain.	*Compression of Brain.*	*Epilepsy.*	*Apoplexy.*	*Hysteria.*	*Fainting.*	*Infantile convulsions.*	*Sun-stroke.*	*Heat-stroke.*	*Shock.*	*Collapse.*
Cause	Blows or falls on head.	Injury to head. Skull often shows signs of injury.	Hereditary predisposition.	Diseased blood vessel bursting in the brain.	People with very nervous temperaments. Excessive joy and sorrow.	Extreme hunger, fatigue. Warm, close or crowded rooms. Loss of blood. Heart-disease.	Teething and bowel troubles.	Exposure to direct rays of sun.	Prolonged exposure to high temperature, *plus* physical exertion.	Severe injuries, *e.g.*, broken bones, burns, etc.	Alcohol, and poisons.
Onset	Sudden	Gradual.	Fits come on without warning.	Sudden ..	Gradual	Gradual	Gradual ..	Gradual ..	Gradual	Gradual ..	Gradual.
Appearance of patient.	Unconscious, but can be roused by shouting.	Deep unconsciousness—Cannot be roused.	Unconscious. Tongue bitten. Bloody froth from mouth.	As in compression of Brain.	Jerky movements of body; patient always sensible.	Unconscious; very pale face and white lips.	Unconscious; cannot be roused. Face muscles twitch.	Unconscious; flushed face.	Slightly unconscious.	Partial insensibility; face pale.	Insensibility varies with amount of alcohol or poison taken.
Eyes	Pupils equal in size and get smaller when exposed to light.	Pupils unequal in size—and are *not* affected by light.	Nothing characteristic.	Do. ..	Eyelids closed, but patient resists opening them.	Nothing characteristic.	Eyelids closed.	Blood-shot; pupils usually contracted.	Dull-looking	Sunken; pupils dilated.	Pupils dilated in alcohol. Pupils contracted in opium.
Breathing ..	Slow and feeble—often hardly perceptible.	Slow, but snorting in character.	At first almost stops, then loud.	Do. ..	Quick	Silent but quick ..	Very quick..	Quick and noisy.	Quiet and easy ..	Very quiet ..	Slow, but snoring in character.
Pulse	Slow and weak ..	Slow and strong.	Quick	Do. ..	Quick	Weak	Quick but weak.	Quick, strong and jumpy.	Quick but feeble ..	Very weak ..	Very weak.
Condition of skin.	Cool	Hot	Not characteristic ..	Do. ..	No change ..	Cool sweat on forehead and palms of hands.	Cold and wet with perspiration.	Very hot and dry; high fever.	Pale and cool ..	Cold and moist.	Cold and moist.
State of muscles.	Lifeless and soft.	One side of body quite limp.	Stiff	Do. ..	False stiffening of muscles.	Slight jerks	Stiff. ..	Trembling, often rigid.	At rest	At rest ..	Quite slack.
Special Treatment.	Head low, absolute rest, warmth to body and limbs.	Dress wound if present.	Place patient so that he cannot injure himself.	Head raised, apply cold.	Cold douche to head, flick face and neck with corner of a wet handkerchief. Keep away sympathetic friends.	Lay flat on back with head low.	Put in hot bath and apply cold to head.	Remove to cool place.	Hot bath	Cover up warmly.	For alcohol, see page 128.
For general treatment, see page 102.	Avoid stimulants	Treat as apoplexy	Place a well-padded piece of wood or a comb between the teeth. After fit encourage natural sleep.	Hot water bottles to feet, mustard poultices to calves of legs.		Give smelling salts or weak ammonia to smell. Give a teaspoonful of sal volatile in a large wineglassful of water to drink.		Pour cold water on head, wrap in sheets wrung out in cold or preferably iced water.	When consciousness returns give stimulants.	Raise foot of bed, and apply hot water bottles. Give hot coffee with plenty of sugar in it, but no alcohol except under medical orders.	For opium, see p. 128. For dhatura, see p. 127. For bhang, see p. 129.

CHAPTER XI.

THE NERVOUS SYSTEM.

THE chief difference between man and the lower animals is the high degree of development of his nervous system, which system consists of two great divisions:

A. The Central or Voluntary System.

B. The Sympathetic or Vegetative System.

A. *The Central Nervous System.*

This consists of :—

1. The Brain.
2. The Spinal Cord or Marrow.
3. The Nerves.

1. *The Brain.*—The brain is enclosed in the skull and consists of a soft greyish-white mass. Its surface is marked by tortuous folds and its structure is most complicated.

It is the seat of the intellect, the will, and the emotions. All the functions of life are under its direct control. Hence the striking difference in its size in man and the lower animals according to their intelligence—in human beings it is one-fortieth of the weight of the body, in the elephant it is one-five hundredth, and in the whale it is one-three thousandth.

2. *The Spinal Cord or Marrow.*—This is a prolongation of the brain which occupies the spinal canal in the backbone. It is a long cylindrical whitish-grey cord and gives off from its side thirty-one pairs of nerves, which go to all parts of the body and preside over movement.

3. *The Nerves.*—These are white cords pearly in appearance which branch off into ever smaller and smaller filaments, the smallest of which can only be seen through the microscope. They extend all over the body, and are necessary to movements, sensation, and nutrition. The whole system of the nerves may be compared to a telegraph department. The brain is the chief office, the sub-offices are in the spinal cord, and the different wires are represented by the nerves. Unlike ordinary telegraph business, however, the messages come and go with almost inconceivable rapidity.

The results of injury to the brain or rupture of blood-vessels into it are :—

(1) Insensibility.
(2) Loss of movement.
(3) Loss of feeling.
(4) Loss of speech.

Where a nerve has been severed as by cutting, shooting or stabbing, loss of feeling and of movement follows. Injuries of the upper part of the spinal cord prove immediately fatal, but injuries lower down only cause paralysis of the lower half of the body.

B. *The Sympathetic Nervous System.*— This system consists of a double chain of small nervous centres which lie along the front of the backbone. They have numerous knotty swellings, and send out numberless delicate branches chiefly to the heart, lungs, stomach, and intestines.

The sympathetic nerves are not subservient to the will, but entirely independent, and control the whole of the functions of organic life, *viz.*, the circulation of the blood, breathing, digestion and excretion. They work steadily on, even when man is asleep or insensible.

There is a large group of these nerves behind the stomach, and it is chiefly due to the effect on them that a kick or blow in the stomach causes such severe symptoms. Shock is chiefly attributable to injury of these nerves.

The following *general rules* for treating insensibility should be committed to memory :—

1. Send for a doctor.
2. Stop bleeding, if present, and examine patient to see if there is a fracture or dislocation before moving him.
3. Place patient in an easy position.
4. Loosen clothing.
5. Give plenty of air.
6. Give nothing by the mouth.
7. Do not leave the patient.
8. Do not presume the patient is drunk, because he smells of alcohol.

The Table on page 98(*a*) shows the causes of the various kinds of insensibility and the means of recognising them.

Shock.

Shock, which has been so frequently referred to, is also called collapse and prostration.

It is a condition of general depression of the whole system and requires special notice. It occurs after severe frights, injuries, and operations. The symptoms are: (1) a weak rapid pulse, (2) paleness of the lips and pinched look on the face, (3) cold and clammy skin, and (4) sometimes there is sickness, but unconsciousness is uncommon.

Treatment.—(1) Place the patient with his head low; (2) cover up with blanket or coat out of doors; if in bed, raise the foot of the bed and apply hot-water bottles and hot blankets; (3) give hot drinks.

CHAPTER XII.

The Organs Concerned in Breathing.

These are :—

1. The windpipe.
2. The bronchial tubes.
3. The lungs.

Breathing or respiration consists of two parts: (1) *inspiration,* the act of drawing air in, and (2) *expiration*, the act of expelling air from, the lungs.

In health, the chest is filled and emptied of air fifteen to eighteen times per minute. The air enters by the nose and mouth and passes *via* the windpipe to the bronchial tubes and lungs.

In the lungs the air gives up oxygen which is its life-giving element to the blood and takes up carbonic acid which is the waste product, the ashes, so to speak, of the lungs.

Air is essential to life, and suspension of breathing is rapidly fatal,

There are many accidents in which the breathing is temporarily suspended.

There are various ways by which the First Aid student can save life by restoring the action of the lungs.

The process of doing so is known as *Artificial Respiration.*

The three varieties and their advantages are given in the following table :—

The Three Methods of Artificial Respiration.

	Schafer's method.	Sylvester's method.	Laborde's method.
1. Clothing of patient.	Waste no time removing clothing.	Remove clothing and ensure absolute freedom of patient's neck, chest and waist.	Remove clothing.
2. Position of patient.	Prone, *i.e.*, back upwards.	Patient flat on his back with a pad placed under shoulder blades.	On back or side.
3. Position of operator.	Kneel at one side, facing patient's head.	Kneel behind patient's head.	Kneel at side of patient.
4. Attention to air passages.	Clear mouth and nostrils of any obstructing material.	Open and wipe mouth and lips of patient. Draw out tongue.	Open and clean mouth.

5. Movements of operator.	Place palms of hands on small of back of patient. Draw forward and slowly apply firm pressure straight downwards upon back and lower part of chest. This excites expiration. Draw your body back and relax pressure but do not remove your hands. This induces inspiration.	(1) Grasp patient's forearms just below the elbow, draw the arms upwards, outwards and towards you with a sweeping movement making the elbows touch the ground. This draws air into the lungs. (2) Bring patient's flexed arms slowly forward, downwards, and inwards, pressing the arms and elbow firmly on chest. This drives air out of the chest.	Seize patient's tongue with a handkerchief and pull it forward. Hold it thus for two seconds, then allow it to recede into the mouth.
6 Auxiliary Efforts.	Smelling salts, Flick chest with damp towel. After treatment, keep patient warm.	Same as for Schafer's method.	Same as for Schafer's method.

The Three Methods of Artificial Respiration—contd.

	Schafer's method.	Sylvester's method.	Laborde's method.
7. Advantages.	Can be very quickly applied by one person.	Well adapted for cases of drowning.	Especially useful when the ribs are broken.

Note.—In all three varieties repeat the procedure fifteen to eighteen times a minute, as this is the number of times a person breathes in health.

ARTIFICIAL RESPIRATION.

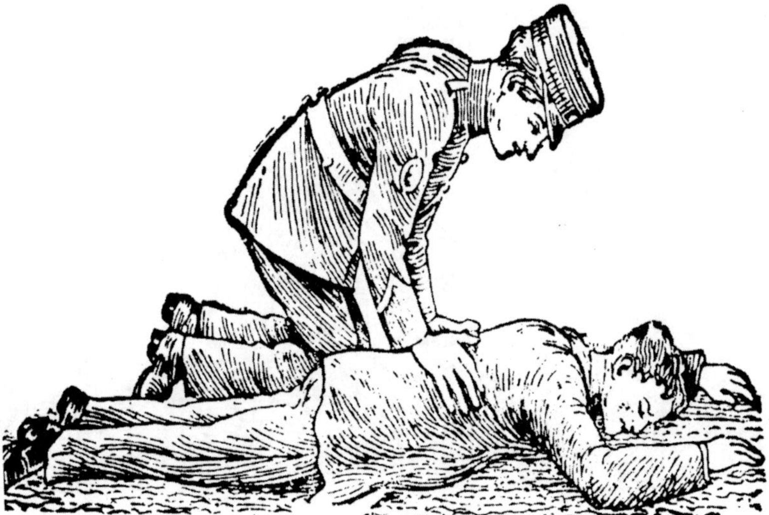

FIG. 43 EXPIRATION.

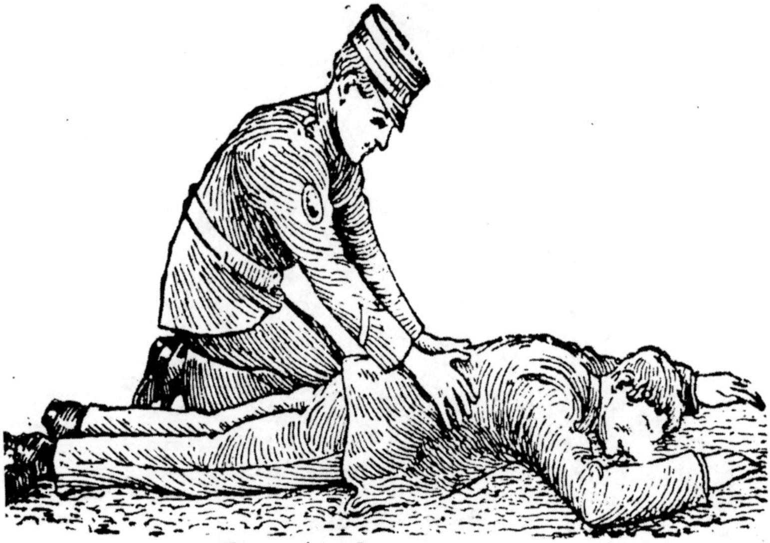

FIG. 44 INSPIRATION.

SCHAFER'S METHOD.

ARTIFICIAL RESPIRATION.

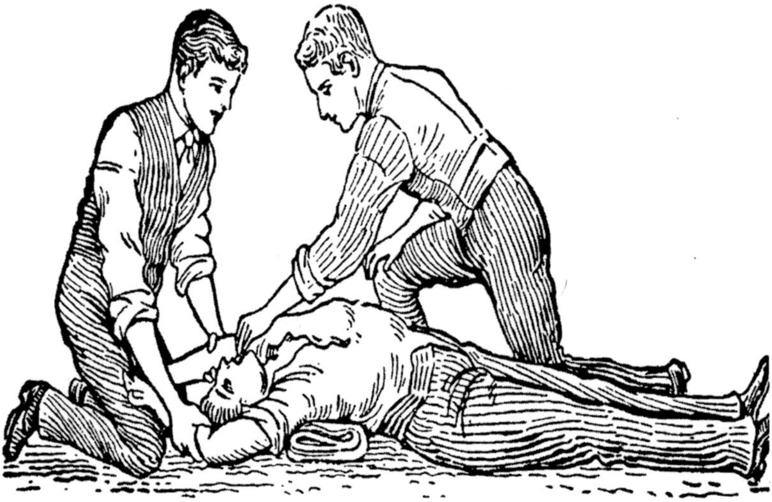

FIG. 45 INSPIRATION.

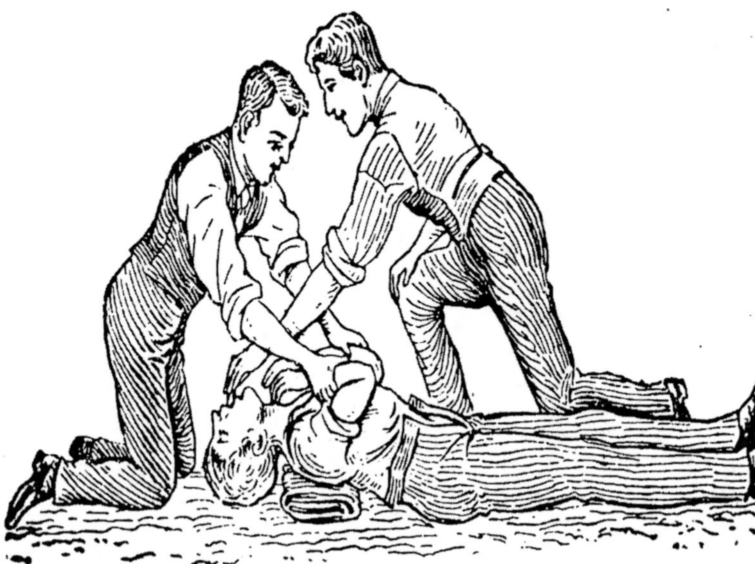

FIG. 46 EXPIRATION.

SYLVESTER'S METHOD.

The following are the chief accidents associated with suspension of breathing :—

1. Hanging.
2. Strangulation.
3. Suffocation.
4. Drowning.
5. Electric Shock.

1. *Hanging—Treatment :—*

(1) Call for help.

(2) Grasp the lower part of the patient.

(3) Raise sufficiently to take the weight of the body off the rope.

(4) Get helper to cut the rope, or release one hand and do it yourself.

(5) Support the body when the rope is cut to prevent it being injured by falling to the ground.

(6) Remove the rope from the neck.

(7) Loosen clothing.

(8) Perform artificial respiration.

2. *Strangulation—Treatment :—*

(1) Remove rope or band round neck.

(2) Loosen clothing.

(3) Open mouth and clean throat.

(4) Perform artificial respiration.

3. *Suffocation.*—This may occur from smoke or gases. The method of rescue from a room full of smoke or gas is similar, *viz.* :—

(1) Tie a handkerchief, folded as a triangular bandage, soaked in water or vinegar and water (1 part of vinegar in four of water) over the face. Bottom edge to be across bridge of nose and point to hang down over the mouth and nose.

(2) Take a few good deep breaths.

(3) Bend low and move quickly to patient's side.

(4) Carry out by fireman's lift.

(5) Perform artificial respiration.

4. *Drowning.*—Death from immersion in water may be caused in many ways besides suffocation,—namely, (1) exhaustion, (2) shock, (3) sudden heart failure, (4) heart disease and many other conditions. This accounts for the fact that strong swimmers often sink at once on falling into the water, without making an attempt to save themselves. Restoration to life by arti-

ficial respiration has occurred where persons have been immersed for as long as a quarter of an hour.

The points to be aimed at in the treatment of a person apparently drowned are :—

(*a*) Removal of obstruction to breathing.

(*b*) Restoration of breathing.

(*c*) Restoration of the body warmth and circulation of the blood.

You must therefore—

(1) Send to the nearest house for blankets, clothing, hot-water bottles, hot tea, hot coffee and stimulants.

(2) Send for a doctor.

(3) Send for a gharrie.

(4) Perform artificial respiration until a doctor pronounces the person dead.

Note—There is no time-limit for carrying out artificial respiration on a person apparently drowned.

Patients have recovered after two or more hours.

When breathing recommences, but not till then, proceed to carry out point (*c*) by means of hot water, hot blankets, hot drinks and stimulants.

5. *Electric Shock.*—The dangers of contact with *bijli* apparatus are now known to the public in a general way.

Contact with an electric cable may produce—

(1) Severe shock.
(2) Insensibility.
(3) Death.

The person is unable to remove the part in contact with the wire as the current deprives him of all power of moving.

Treatment.—The first essential is: (*a*) to switch off the electrical current if possible; (*b*) if this is impracticable or likely to cause serious delay, to get the sufferer away from the wire; but the person rendering First Aid must understand that he does so at great risk of being himself affected by the current. The rescuer must, what is called, insulate himself from the current, that is use a substance for touching the patient through which electricity cannot readily pass. Such substances are:—

1. India-rubber articles.
2. Dry wood.

3. Dry glass.
4. Dry straw.
5. Dry cloth.

All the common metals, such as iron, copper, brass, etc., allow electricity to pass freely and must be avoided. Water is also a good conductor, and in dealing with electric shock damp clothing increases the risk of the rescuer.

Proceed therefore as follows :—

(1) Shove the person away from contact with the cable by means of a dry pole ; or

(2) Push him away with the sleeve of a dry coat or an empty India-rubber tobacco pouch used as a glove ; or

(3) Throw a dry coat held by the sleeves, or a dry belt or puttee over the head or round the body of the victim and drag him away from contact.

(4) After rescuing the patient carry out the general treatment for insensibility.

(5) Perform artificial respiration if breathing has ceased.

(6) Treat shock.

(7) Dress burns.

Choking.—If a person swallows a bone

or anything, which obstructs the windpipe, open the mouth and pass the forefinger right to the back of the throat and try to get out the article which is causing the mischief.

If the finger induces vomiting, so much the better; should this fail, place the head well forward and thump the back well between the shoulder-blades. It is sometimes useful to make the patient run a short distance, in doing which the body may be expelled.

CHAPTER XIII.

POISONS AND THEIR TREATMENT.

A poison is a substance which, when taken into the mouth or stomach or when absorbed into the blood, is capable of seriously affecting health or destroying life.

Poisoning is much more frequent in India than in Europe, and the subject is consequently dealt with more fully in this *Manual* than in English text-books of First Aid.

Generally speaking, poisoning may be suspected by: (1) the sudden appearance of alarming symptoms in a person in good health, (2) the onset of the symptoms soon after food or drink has been taken.

The symptoms vary in character, and the reatment depends on the poison taken.

You must not at once assume that a person who is suffering from sudden distressing symptoms has been poisoned. One man's meat is another man's poison, and occasionally apparently sound food may cause signs of poisoning in some of the persons who have consumed it and not in others. Unsound foods may, as will be seen in the following Table (p. 124,) produce the conditions known as ptomaine poisoning and not infrequently cause death.

When called to render First Aid in a case of suspected poisoning: (1) Take a quick glance round the room or vicinity to endeavour to detect a bottle denoting the poison which has been swallowed. (2) Throw nothing whatsoever away. (3) Carefully note any stains on the mouth or the clothes. These are usually present when corrosive poisons have been taken; and modify the treatment. (4) Note the odour of the breath which will be important in carbolic acid, prussic acid, opium and alcoholic poisoning. (5) Note the presence or absence of drowsiness. (6) Observe the state of the pupils, which are dilated in *dhatura* and contracted in opium poisoning.

The General Treatment of Poisons.—The First Aid treatment of poisons is :—(1) Send for Medical help, informing the doctor of the poison suspected. (2) Endeavour to neutralise and dilute the poison. (3) Protect the internal surface of the stomach and bowels by giving olive, vegetable or animal oil, milk, white of eggs, strong tea or flour and water. (4) *Emetics must only be given when there are no stains on the mouth or lips.* The most efficient means of producing vomiting is two tablespoonfuls of mustard, or a tablespoonful of salt, to a tumbler of lukewarm water.

Poisons may be grouped according to their action as :—

1. Narcotics, *i.e.*, sleep-producing.
2. Irritants, such as the metallic poisons, arsenic and mercury, powdered glass, and kerosine oil.
3. Corrosive, *i.e.*, substances which destroy the tissues, such as the strong acids.
4. Nerve poisons, *i.e.*, substances which act chiefly on the nerves, producing delirium or great excitement, such as belladonna, alcohol, Indian hemp, mushrooms, etc.

As in India persons are frequently far from medical aid, it is thought that the following table which indicates in simple language the treatment of all the principal poisons will be found acceptable in the Indian household :—

The commoner forms of Poisoning, their recognition and treatment.

	Poisons.	Symptoms.	Treatment.
Corrosives:	Acids such as sulphuric & nitric acids & spirit of salts.	(1) Lips and mouth stained either white (spirit of salts), yellowish (nitric acid), or black (sulphuric acid). (2) Pain in mouth, throat and belly. (3) Intense thirst. (4) Blood-coloured vomit. (5) Difficulty in talking. (6) Collapse.	(1) Avoid emetics; (2) Give a tablespoonful of bicarbonate of soda or chalk, well mixed in half a pint of water. (3) Follow this with olive oil (¼ pint in one pint of water.) (4) Give milk freely.
	Carbolic Acid.	(1) Lips and mouth stained white. (2) Muscles soft and useless.	Give— (1) Epsom salts or sulphate of soda, half an ounce in half a pint of warm water.

The commoner forms of Poisoning, their recognition and treatment—contd.

	Poisons.	Symptoms.	Treatment.
Corrosives.		(3) Collapse. (4) Carbolic acid smell from breath.	(2) Olive oil ($\frac{1}{4}$ pint to one pint water). (3) Milk freely. (4) Alcohol freely. (5) Warmth to feet. (6) Artificial respiration.
	Strong alkalies such as ammon i a, and caustic soda and potash.	(1) Purging and vomiting (always present.) (2) Pain and straining. (3) Collapse.	(1) Avoid emetics. Give— (2) Vinegar or lemon or lime juice diluted with water freely. (3) Milk freely. (4) Olive oil ($\frac{1}{4}$ pint to one pint water.)

	Poison	Symptoms	Treatment
Irritants.	Arsenic.	(1) Continual vomiting and purging, (2) Cramps and pains in calves of legs. (3) Patient exhausted and insensible. *N.B.—Arsenic poisoning very much resembles cholera.*	(1) Encourage rapid vomiting by lukewarm salt and water. (2) Milk, brandy and olive oil. (3) Artificial respiration and warmth to feet.
	Powdered glass.	(1) Very severe pain in stomach. (2) This is a mechanical poison, which produces (*a*) pain in the stomach, (*b*) diarrhœa, (*c*) straining with blood in the stools, and (*d*) sometimes vomiting ; the vomitted matter contains particles of the powdered glass which may be seen with a hand lens.	(1) First give large quantities of bulky food, such as bread, potatoes and rice to mix with the glass and protect the walls of the stomach against it—then an emetic.
	Kerosine oil.	(1) Burning pain in mouth and throat.	(1) Emetic. (2) Brandy.

The commoner forms of Poisoning, their recognition and treatment—contd.

	Poisons.	Symptoms.	Treatment.
Irritants.		(2) Vomited mater shows oily substance and smells of kerosine. (3) Breath smells of kerosine. (4) Intense thirst. (5) Collapse and insensibility..	(3) Warmth to feet.
	Ptomaines *i.e.* *Meat poisons.* *Fish poisons.*	(1) Vomiting and purging. (2) Great exhaustion and muscular weakness. (3) Tongue brown coloured. (4) Fever and quick pulse. *N.B.—Resembles cholera, but fever is never present in cholera.*	(1) Emetics. (2) Castor oil, two ounces. (3) Brandy and hot milk. (4) Warmth to feet. (5) Artificial respiration.
	Phosphorus; this poison is contained in many rat	(1) Pain and vomiting; vomited matter smells of garlic, and may be luminous in the dark.	(1) Emetics.

Irritants,	poisons and in matches.	(2) Bleeding from nose. (3) Convulsions.	(2) Permanganate of potash, five grains in a pint of water. (3) Stimulants. (4) Avoid oils.
	Mercury.	(1) Metallic taste in mouth. (2) Vomiting and purging. (3) Tongue whitish. (4) Collapse.	(1) Flour and water. (2) Then emetic, such as common salt in warm water. (3) Lemonade and brandy.
	Turpentine.	(1) Breathing snoring in character. (2) Pupils small. (3) Muscles jerky and stiff. (4) Turpentine odour from breath and smell of violets from urine.	(1) Emetics. (2) Purgatives. (3) Demulcent drinks such as milk and flour and water.

*The commoner forms of **Poisoning**, their recognition and treatment*—contd.

	Poisons.	Symptoms.	Treatment.
Narcotics.	Opium and its preparations which are very numerous and include laudanum, morphia, chlorodyne and paregoric.	(1) Drowsiness. (2) *Pupils very small* (pin-point in size). (3) Partial insensibility but can be roused. (4) Breathing slow and deep. (5) Skin covered with clammy sweat. (6) Then collapse. (7) *Breath smells of opium.*	(1) Induce vomiting by salt and water. (2) Give large draughts of hot tea. (3) Permanganate of potash solution, 10 grains to pint of water. (4) Keep patient roused by slapping him on the face and body with a wet towel and walking him about occasionally. (5) Artificial respiration.

Nerve Poisons.			
	Belladonna	Same symptoms as *Dhatura*.	Same treatment as *Dhatura*.
	Dhatura is one of the commonest Indian poisons.	(1) Dryness of throat. (2) Difficulty of swallowing and thirst. (3) Giddiness and staggering. (4) Flushed face. (5) Pupils enlarged. (6) Patient wanders about, talks wildly, is easily intimidated, grasps at imaginary objects and picks at his clothes. From this boisterous stage he becomes insensible and exhausted.	(1) Emetics, *e.g.*, common salt in warm water. (2) Stimulants, *e.g.*, brandy. (3) Hot tea or coffee. (4) Artificial respiration. (5) Hot water bottles and friction to the limbs.
	Prussic Acid and Cyanide of Potassium.	(1) The symptoms come on immediately. (2) Giddiness and staggering. (3) Patient falls insensible. (4) Breathing very distressed and gasping. (5) Eyes shining and bright and pupils enlarged. (6) Collapse. (7) Smell of bitter almonds from breath.	(1) Carry patient into open air if possible. (2) Dash cold water to face and back. (3) Artificial respiration. 4) Smelling salts to nostrils. (5) Hot tea.

The commoner forms of Poisoning, their recognition and treatment—contd.

	Poisons.	Symptoms.	Treatment.
Nerve Poisons.			*N.B.—This poison acts very rapidly, therefore be prompt in treatment.*
	Alcohol.	(1) Flushed face and red eyes. (2) Lips bluish. (3) Giddiness and staggering walk. (4) Insensibility (variable). (5) Smell of liquor from breath.	(1) Rouse patient by dashing cold water in his face. (2) Emetic when conscious. (3) Hot tea. (4) Artificial respiration. (5) Smelling salts to nostrils.
	Cocaine.	(1) Patient pale and faint. (2) Skin dry. (3) Pulse and breathing quick.	(1) Emetics, *e.g.*, common salt in water.

		(4) Tremor of muscles. (5) Insensibility.	(2) Brandy. (3) Artificial respiration.
Nerve Poisons.	Mushrooms and Poisonous Fungi.	(1) Thirst and pain in belly. (2) Vomiting and purging. (3) Patient sometimes boisterous at first, then quiet. (4) Breathing is snoring in character. (5) Enlarged pupils. Insensibility.	(1) Emetics. (2) Purgative, *e.g.*, castor oil two ounces. (3) Brandy. (4) Warmth to extremities.
	Indian Hemp; known popularly as *B h a n g* (*leaves*). *Gunja* (*flowering tops*) *and Charas* (*resinous extract*).	(1) Patient at first boisterous, during this stage he may either laugh, sing or exhibit much excitement. (2) Then he becomes drowsy and insensible. (3) Pupils enlarged.	(1) Emetic. (2) Hot tea. (3) Warmth to feet. (4) Artificial respiration.

	Poisons.	Symptoms.	Treatment.
Nerve Poisons.	Strychnine & Nux-vomica, *this poison is contained in some vermin killers.*	(1) Violent convulsions and arching of the back. (2) Lock-jaw. (3) Eyeballs prominent and pupils dilated. (4) Difficulty in breathing. (5) Pulse feeble and rapid.	(1) Emetics. (2) Ten grains of permanganate of potash in a pint of hot water. (3) Stronger tea or coffee. (4) A Surgeon will give chloroform. (5) Artificial respiration, which however is usually only possible under chloroform.

CHAPTER XIV.

THE DIGESTIVE SYSTEM AND THE EYE, EAR AND NOSE.

The Digestive System consists of :—

1. The Mouth and Throat.
2. The Stomach.
3. The Bowels or Intestines.
4. The Liver.
5. The Pancreas or Sweetbread.

This system is of the utmost importance to the individual, but of less importance to the renderer of First Aid than any other part of the body. It only concerns him in connection with a variety of "so-called strain" which occurs chiefly in the region of the groin and is known as—

Rupture or Hernia.—In this case one of the contents of the abdomen, usually the bowel, protrudes through the wall of the belly beneath the skin. The most common situation is just below the groin in women and just above it in men.

In these situations it forms a soft, more or less rounded, swelling which generally disappears when the patient lies down.

A rupture usually gives no symptoms until for some reason the portion of the intestine, which it consists of, becomes nipped in the aperture through which it protrudes. This is a very serious condition.

The Symptoms and Signs of "nipped" or Strangulated Rupture are—

(1) Sensation by the patient of something having given way.
(2) Pain, which may be very acute.
(3) Swelling, usually in the groin.
(4) Relief on bending the knee.
(5) Sometimes vomiting.

Treatment :—

(1) Send for medical help.
(2) Make the patient lie down.
(3) Raise the head and body and bend the legs on the thigh.
(4) Apply ice or cold water dressing to the part.

The Eye.

Foreign Body in the Eye.—A. When beneath the Lower Lid.—It is easy enough to remove a foreign body if it settles under the lower lid by the following method: (1) place the thumb below the lower lid and pull it downwards. (2) Wet the corner of a clean handkerchief or clean rag and wipe out the offending body.

B. When beneath Upper Lid.—A good plan is to pull the upper eyelid forward and downward by grasping the lashes between the finger and thumb and directing the patient to look upward. In this way the lashes of the lower lid sweep the inside of the upper lid and remove the foreign body. If this device does not remove the offending material send for a doctor, but if one is not available, the upper lid can be explored by placing a match, tooth-pick or similar small rod against the lid, grasping the lashes and pulling them upwards over the rod. The eyelid turns inside out, like a pocket, and the foreign body can then be seen and easily removed.

If lime or a sharp splinter enters the eye, a doctor should be immediately sent for, but while waiting for him drop in one or two drops of castor-oil which gives much relief

The Ear.

Foreign Body in the Ear.—Children love to insert peas and all sorts of articles into various cavities of the body, the ear being the favourite. This is an unfortunate practice as it is very dangerous. Parents must never attempt to remove these articles themselves, but must always send for a doctor ; if, however, an earwig or other insect enters the ear, pour salad or any vegetable oil that is handy into the ear and it will float the insect out almost immediately.

The Nose.

Foreign Body in the Nose.—Induce sneezing by giving the patient a pinch of pepper or snuff, or try to get the body out by gentle syringing, but if such efforts fail, medical aid should be sought. Foreign bodies in the nose are not immediately dangerous and rarely do any serious mischief before they have received attention from a surgeon.

The First Aider must on no account attempt to extract foreign bodies from the ear or the nose with a hairpin or other implement.

CHAPTER XV.

Improvised Method of Carrying the Injured or Sick.

These vary according to the number of persons available to carry the patient.

A. Carrying by One Person :—

The following four methods are available :—

1. The Friend's Grip.
2. Pick-a-back.
3. The Back Lift.
4. The Fireman's Lift.

1.—*The Friend's Grip.*—This can only be used to help a person with an injury to one lower limb other than a broken bone, such as a sprained ankle or crushed foot. The bearer stands close to the patient on the same side as the injury, and (1) brings the patient's arm round his neck, (2) seizes the patient's wrist with one hand, (3) passes the other arm round the patient's waist, (4) the patient bends the knee of the injured side to keep the foot off the ground, and hops whilst the bearer walks.

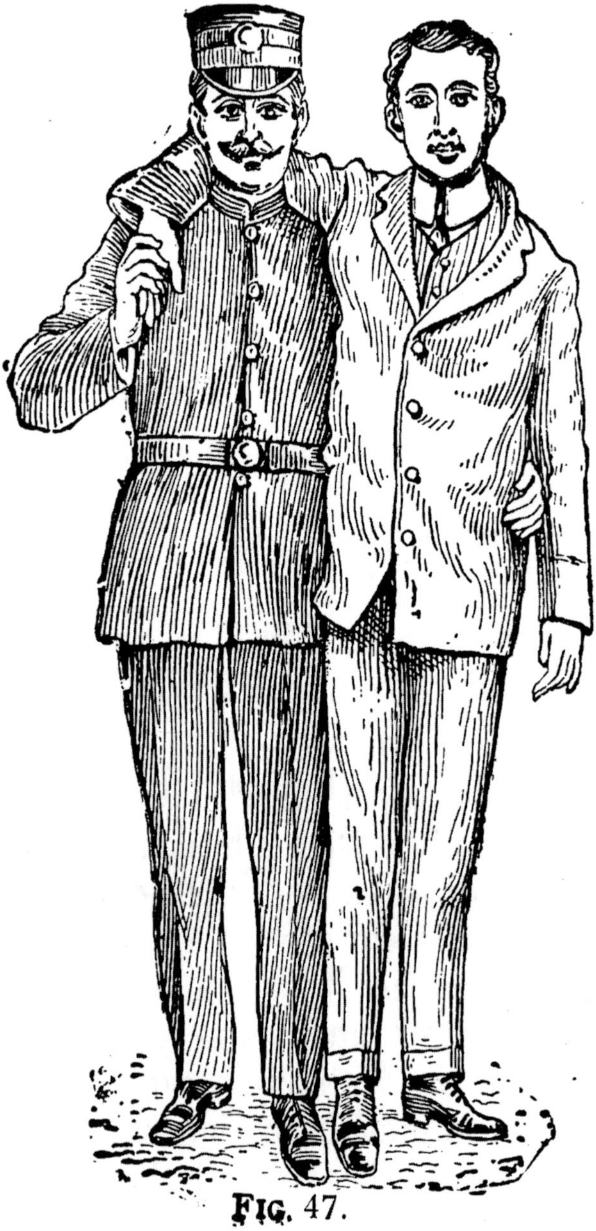

FIG. 47.

THE FRIEND'S GRIP.

The bearer is sometimes recommended to stand on the opposite side to the injured limb ; this is not advisable.

2.—*Pick-a-back.*—The injured person may be carried pick-a-back if his injury permits.

3.—*The Back Lift.*—If the patient is able to stand, place him with his back to yours, then (1) slightly stoop, (2) place your hands over your shoulders, (3) grasp the patient under the arm-pits, (4) bring his weight well up into the small of the back, and (5) stand up. To lower the patient to the ground sink down on the left knee and place him in a sitting posture.

4.—*The Fireman's Lift.*—This is especially suitable in cases of insensibility. The patient is lifted on to the shoulder in the following manner : (1) Roll the patient over on his face and bring his arms to the sides, (2) kneel down with one knee on either side of the patient's head, pass your hands, palms uppermost, beneath his arm-pits, and raise him on his knees, (3) move your arms gradually downwards until they encircle the patient's waist, clasping the hands over the small of the back, and raise him on to his feet, (4) grasp the patient's right wrist with your left hand, and place his right arm round your neck. Stoop until your right shoulder is opposite his right groin, and at the same time pass your right hand round his thigh and bring his weight well on the centre of your back, (5) transfer the patient's right wrist from your left to your right hand, and stand up.

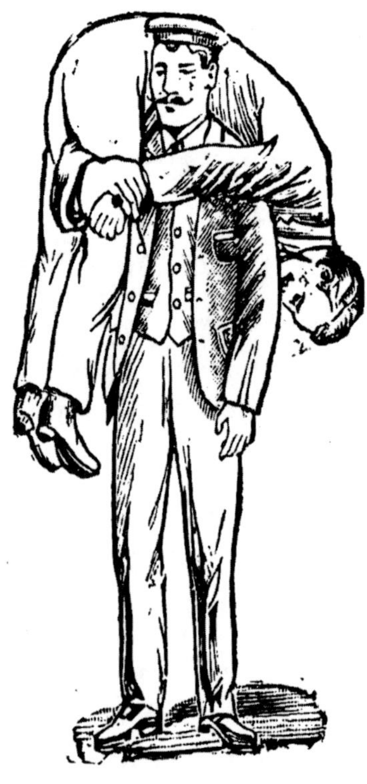

FIG. 48.—FIREMAN'S LIFT.

B. Carriage by Two Persons :—

The following methods are available :—

1. The Fore and Aft Method.
2. Hand Seats
3. Improvised Stretchers.

1. *The Fore and Aft Method.*—This method can only be used for a person not seriously injured. If the person has to be carried a long way, an improvised chair stretcher is always preferable.

The method is applied as follows :—

(1) One man stands behind the injured person and passes his hands and forearms beneath the patient's arm-pits, (2) the second turns his back to the patient and steps between his legs, he then stoops down and grasps the patient's knees from the outside, (3) both bearers now stand up, lifting the patient.

The Chair Stretcher.—A chair can be converted into a stretcher for sitting-up cases by lashing poles or lathis beneath the seat (Fig. 49.)

2. *Hand Seats.*—This method of carrying is only suited for moderate injuries where stretchers are not available.

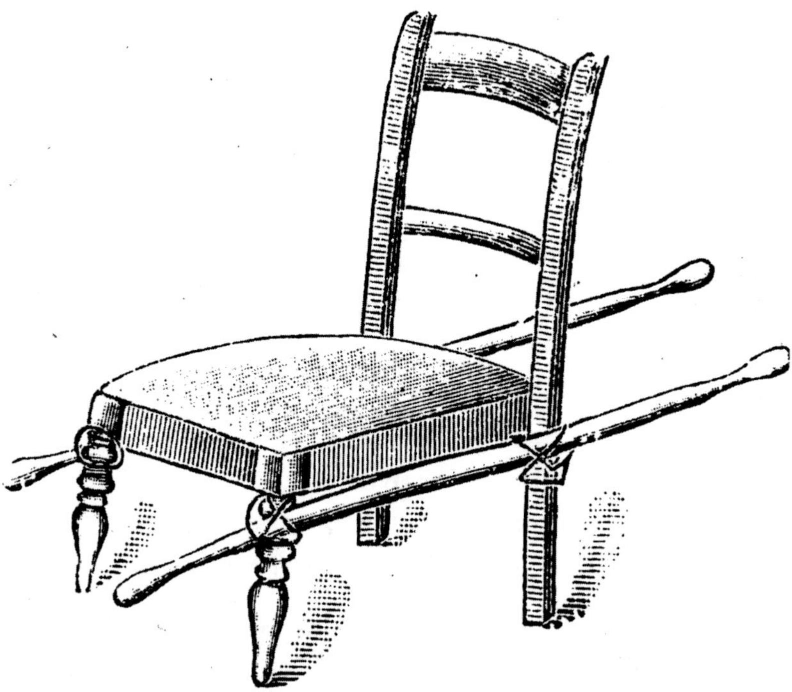

FIG. 49.—CARRYING CHAIR.

There are three varieties, *viz.*;—

(1) Two-Handed Seats.

(2) Three-Handed Seats.

(3) Four-Handed Seats.

(1) *The Two-Handed Seat.*—The hands to form this seat may be grasped in two ways.

(*a*) *The "clasp-hand" or "prayer grip."*—The bearers face each other. Opposite hands are presented to each other, palms upwards, the fingers straight and spread out. The fingers are interlocked and the hands clasped. The palms of the hands thus clasped should be brought together to prevent strain on the fingers.

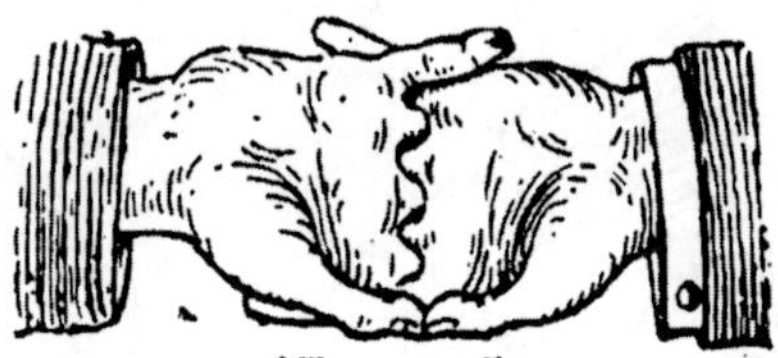

FIG. 50.

CLASP-HANDED SEAT.

(*b*) *The "Hook-Grip."*—Each bearer bends his fingers at the second joint, one bearer with back of the hand uppermost, the other with back of the hand downwards. The bent fingers are hooked together. A handkerchief between the fingers eases the

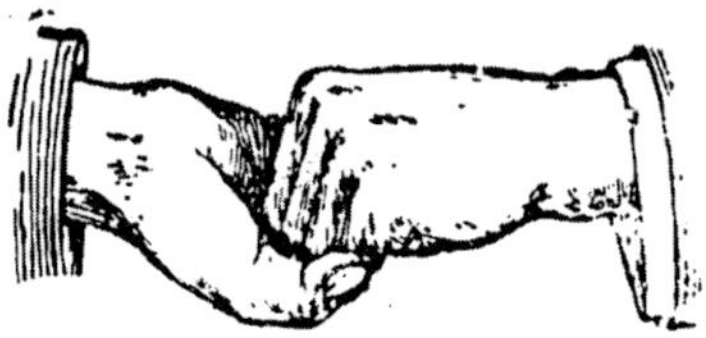

FIG. 51.
HOOK-GRIP.

strain on the fingers, or gloves may be worn, which have the same effect. Having prepared the two-handed seat, the bearers stoop down behind the patient as shown in Fig. 52 and carry him as shown in Fig. 53.

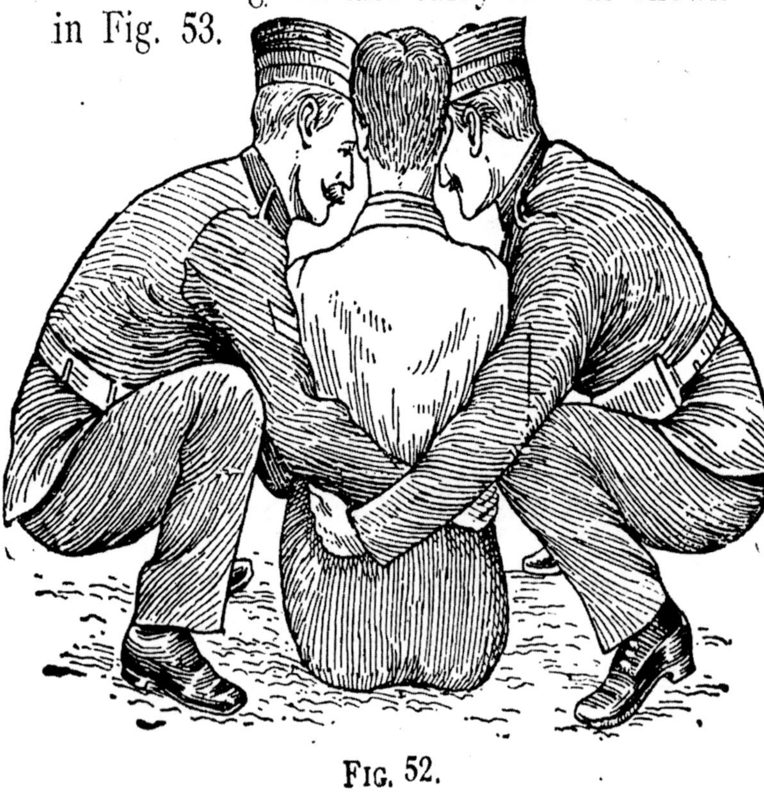

FIG. 52.

LIFTING BY TWO-HANDED SEAT

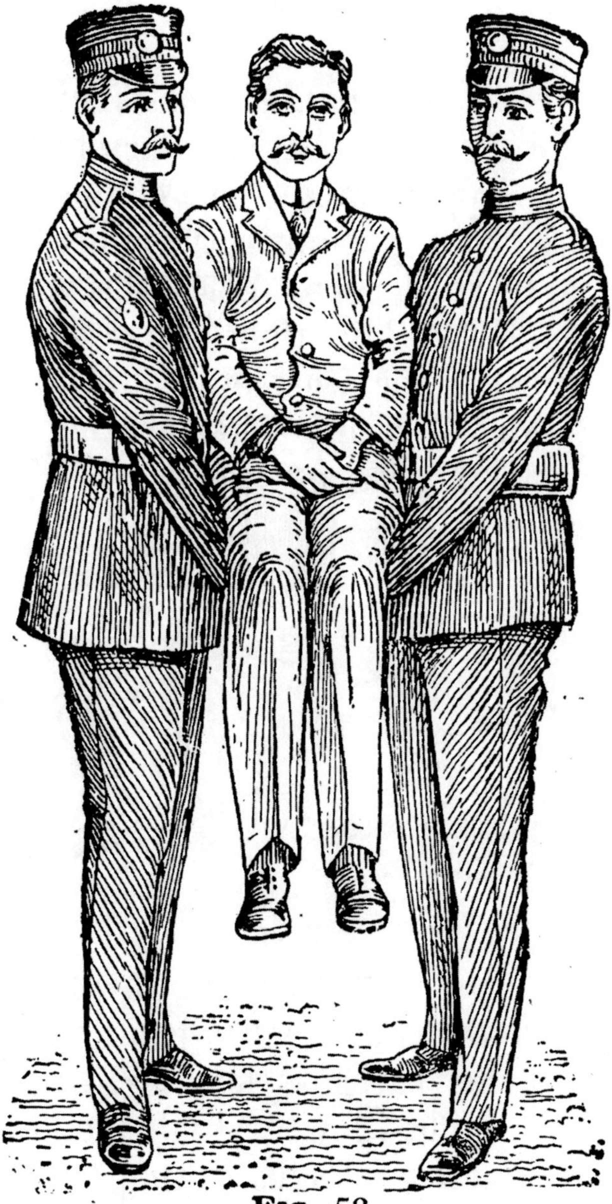

Fig. 53.

Carrying by Two-Handed Seat.

(2) *The Three-Handed Seat.*—This seat is useful for carrying a patient when he is able to use his upper limbs. One of the bearers has a free hand to support an injured lower limb. (2) No. 1 bearer grasps his own left forearm with his right hand, and the right wrist of the other bearer with his left hand. No. 2 bearer grasps the No. 1 bearer's right wrist with his right hand.

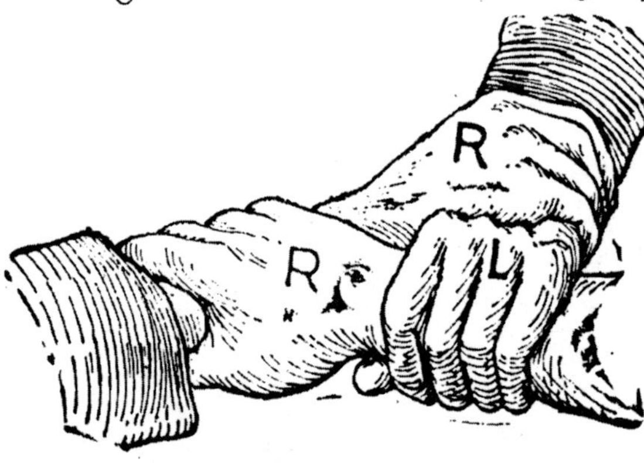

FIG. 54.

GRIP FOR THREE-HANDED SEAT.

This leaves his left hand free to support the patient's left leg. For the patient's right lower limb follow the same directions, substituting "right" for "left" and "left" for "right." The bearers stoop down. (2) The patient passes an arm round the neck of each bearer, sits on the seat and is raised from the ground by the bearers. (3) The bearers rise together.

(3) *The Four-Handed Seat.*—Each bearer seizes his own left wrist with his right hand and, bringing the hands together, each grasps the opposite bearer's right wrist.

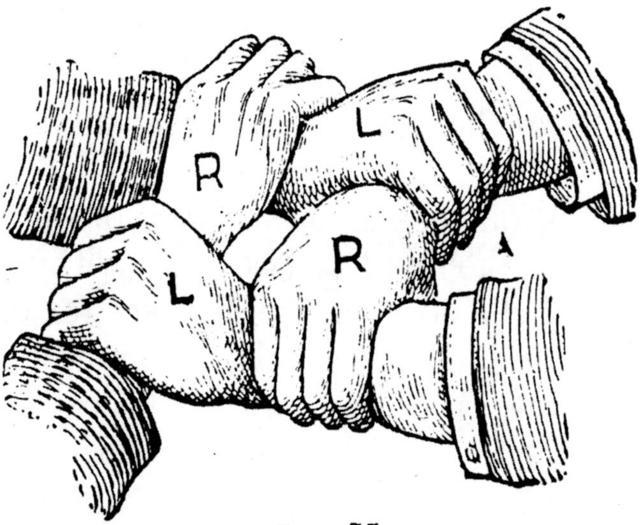

FIG 55.

GRIP FOR FOUR-HANDED SEAT.

In carrying patients by hand seats the bearers move by a side step.

C. *Carriage by Three or More Persons.*—The best method where a dhoolie is not available is some form of improvised stretcher.

In India a wounded or injured person is usually carried on a charpoy which has, however, the following serious disadvantages :—

1. It is cumbersome.
2. It sags.
3. The patient must usually be removed before he can be taken into a house or placed in a wagon.

If possible, it is therefore always advisable to improvise a stretcher.

This can be done in the following simple way :—

Spread out a blanket, a piece of dhurrie, or a horse jhool. Lay two poles within two inches of the edges of the blanket (or other article) and fold the blanket round the poles ; roll up in this way until a bed of 20 to 22 inches breadth is left between them. If only two bearers are available, the unfolded material must be stitched by a packing or improvised needle to the blanket bed, and the breadth maintained by an improvised cross-bar at each end. If no means of stitching by a needle are to hand, holes may be made in the blankets and twine or thin rope passed through and tied off so as to fix the blanket, jhool, or dhurrie firmly on the poles.

Carrying Stretchers over Obstacles.—As a rule, stretchers should not be carried over obstacles, but in preference a detour should be made. A gap should be chosen in preference to passing the stretcher over walls, and a bridge in preference to conveyance over nullahs or streams. When these obstacles cannot be avoided, the following method should be adopted :—

1. *Walls.*—One bearer should stand at each corner of the stretcher. The stretcher should be raised and the front part placed on the top of the wall. Two bearers then climb over the wall, and the stretcher is passed gently forward until the end only rests on the wall. The remaining bearers then climb over and the stretcher is lifted from the wall and placed on the ground, and the bearers lift it as in stretcher drill.

2. *Nullahs.*—The stretcher is placed on the ground at one side of the nullah. One bearer crosses to the opposite bank. Two bearers enter the nullah and support the stretcher as it is passed by the fourth bearer.

When the handles reach the bearer on the opposite bank, the bearers pass the stretcher over the nullah. When it arrives on the opposite bank, the last bearer crosses and falls into place with the other bearers at the stretcher.

CHAPTER XVI.

STRETCHER DRILL.

Stretcher.

The parts of a stretcher are twelve in number, *viz.*, 2 poles, 2 traverses, 4 rollers or

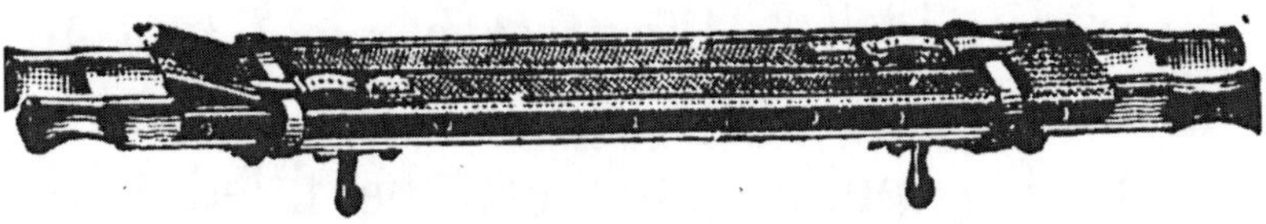

FIG. 56.—ORDINARY STRETCHER—CLOSED.

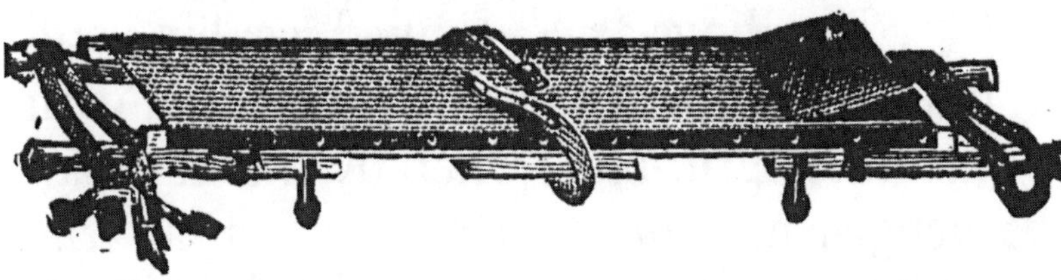

FIG. 57.—TELESCOPIC-HANDLED STRETCHER—OPEN.

runners, 1 pillow sack, 2 shoulder slings, and the stretcher bed.

The St. John Stretcher :—

(1) The poles are either square with rounded handles, and measure 7 feet 9 inches, or are made with telescopic handles to measure, when closed, only six feet.

(2) The traverses are the metal jointed bars on the under surface to keep the poles apart and the canvas taut when the stretcher is opened.

(3) The rollers are small gunmetal wheels or shaped pieces of metal for sliding the stretcher along the bottom of a wagon.

(4) The canvas bed is 6 feet in length and the total width of the stretcher is 1 foot 10 inches.

(5) The pillow sack can be filled with straw, hay, or clothing to form a pillow.

(6) The slings are of tanned webbing and at one end of the sling is a loop provided with a buckle or grip-plate whereby the sling can be lengthened or shortened, and at the opposite end is a transverse leather strap with buckle used to fit around the stretcher when closed.

(7) The weight of the Service stretcher is 34 lbs., but the St. John Ambulance pattern only weighs 22 lbs.

The following is the Military stretcher drill adapted for use by Ambulance units.

(2) *Formation of Stretcher Squads.*

Previous to the parade, the stretchers will be laid in a heap on the ground.

The detachment will be drawn up in single rank, sized, dressed and numbered as follows :—

Sizing the Bearers.

Tallest on the Right, Shortest on the Left, in Single Rank,—Size. The whole will break off and arrange themselves according to their size in single rank, the tallest on the right and shortest on the left, and take up their dressing by the right.

Number. The bearers will number consecutively from right to left.

Odd Numbers One Pace Forward, Even Numbers One Pace Step Back,—March. The odd numbers will take one pace forward, and the even numbers will step back one pace.

Number One Stand Fast, Ranks, Right and Left Turn. The odd numbers, with the exception of Number One, will turn to the right, the even numbers to the left.

Form Company, Quick—March. The whole will step off, the even numbers wheeling round to the right and following the left-hand man of the odd numbers. No. 3 will form up two paces in rear of No. 1, No. 5 on the left of No. 1, No. 7 in rear of No. 5, No. 9 on the left of No. 5; and so on. The leading men of the even numbers will always form in the rear rank and the next man in the front rank. As the men arrive in their places they will turn to the left, and take up their dressing.

FORMING THE SQUADS.

"*By Fours, Number.*"—The front rank number by fours from the right, commencing at No. 1, the bearers calling out 1, 2, 3, 4; 1, 2, and so on. Nos. 1, 5, 9, 13 of the front and rear ranks of original alignment thus become Nos. 1 of squads (Fig. 58*a*).

Squads "at the Halt, Left Form—Quick March—Right Turn."—No. 4 of each squad in front rank turns to his left, the remaining bearers of front rank make a partial turn to the left. The rear rank remain steady (Fig. 58*b*). On the word "March," the whole, except No. 4, who stands steady, step off to their places in the new alignment (Fig. 58*c*); on the word "Turn," all turn to the right.

The bearers are now in fours (stretcher squads.)

"*Right Dress.*"—No. 1 of right squad remains steady, the remaining No. 1 bearers each take up position one pace from and in line with the bearers on the right; the other bearers (Nos. 2, 3, and 4) place themselves one pace in the rear of and covering the bearer in front of them (that is, 2 covers 1, 3 covers 2, and 4 covers 3 in each squad) (Fig. 58*d.*)

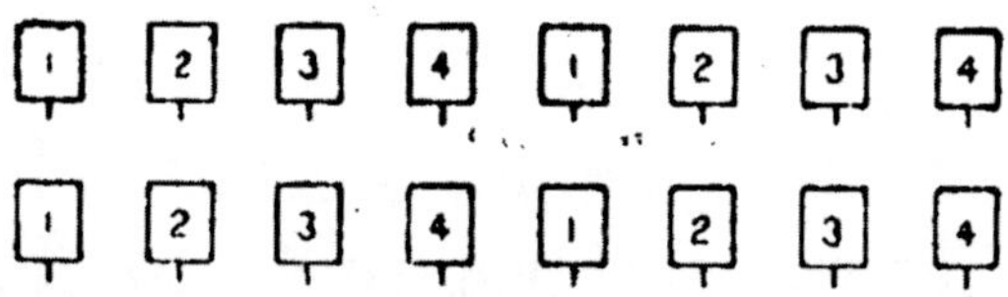

FIG. 58*a*.—BY SQUADS—NUMBER.

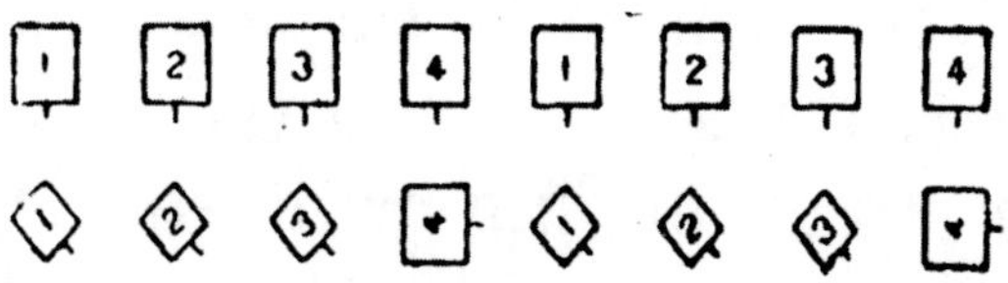

FIG. 58*b*.
SQUADS AT THE HALT—LEFT FORM.

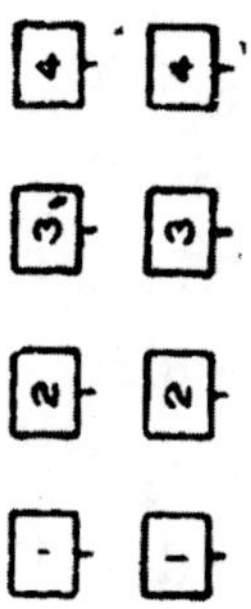

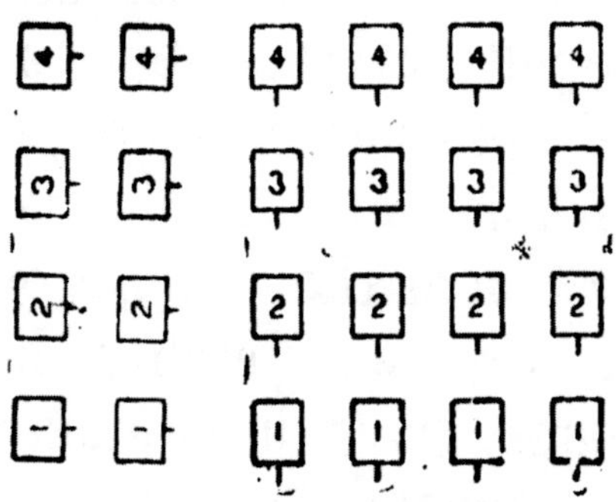

FIG. 58*c*.—MARCH. FIG. 58*d*. RIGHT TURN—RIGHT DRESS.

FIG. 58.—FORMATION OF SQUADS.

Supplying Stretchers.

The squads having been formed, the next step is to begin stretcher drill.

"*No. 3 Bearers—Right (or Left) Turn—Supply Stretchers—Quick March.*"—

At the word, "March," the No. 3 bearers, with or without a guide (corporal) in charge, march by the shortest route to the pile of stretchers, where each bearer in turn lays hold of the handle at the head end of the stretcher, raises it to a perpendicular position in front of him with the left hand, rollers (or U-shaped bracket) to the front, stoops, grasping the lower rollers with his right hand, places the stretcher on his right shoulder at the slope, and rising to the erect position, leads on, stepping shorter or marking time, until the others are ready. As soon as the last bearer has provided himself with a stretcher, he, or the guide in charge, gives the command "About Turn." The whole turn about and rejoin their squads in quick time, halting at the command "Halt" from the guide (or without further word of command if no guide is present) as they arrive in their places, when the instructor or section commander gives the command "Left (or Right) Turn," and the No. 3 bearers turn in the direction named. The lower handles of the stretchers are then placed on the ground, and the stretcher is held perpendicularly.

"*Lower Stretchers.*"—The No. 3 bearers place the stretchers on the ground to the right of the squads, by passing the lower handles (foot of stretcher) forward, rollers to the right, front end of the poles (foot of stretchers) in line with the toes of Nos. 1, and rise together, working by the right.

"*Stand to Stretchers.*"—On the words "Stretchers," the Nos. 1 place themselves with their toes in line with the front end of the pole, Nos. 3 with their heels in line with the rear end of the pole, allowing sufficient room for turning. Nos. 2 take position at centre of poles, Nos. 1, 2 and 3 bearers thus standing on the left of the stretcher. Each No. 4

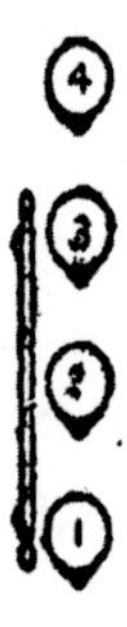

FIG. 59.—STAND TO STRETCHERS.

bearer will take up position one pace in rear of and covering the bearer (No. 3) in front of him (Fig. 59).

PREPARING AND CLOSING STRETCHERS.

The preparing of stretchers is only performed in extended order, that is, with an interval of four paces between each stretcher squad. To arrange the bearers in this position the word of command is: *From the Left (or Right) to four paces—Extend.* On the word *Extend*, the named squad stands fast (or if on the move continues to move on in quick time). The remainder march (or double) to their places and turn on to their front, taking up their dressing by the directing flank. On the commencement of the movement No. 4 places himself on the right of the stretcher.

"*Prepare Stretchers.*"—The No. 4 bearers on the right of the stretchers take a side pace of 30 (or two side paces of 15) inches to the right, Nos. 1 and 3 then turn to the right, kneel on the left knee, unbuckle the transverse straps and drop the slings upon the ground, separate the poles and straighten the traverse; each now takes up a sling, doubles it on itself, slips the loop thus formed on the near handle, grip-plate (buckle) uppermost.

Taking the time from the right they rise, and turn to the left together.

"*Close Stretchers.*"—Nos. 1 and 3 turn to the right, kneel on the left knee, remove the slings and place them on the ground beside them, push in the traverse, raise the canvas, and bring the poles together.

Taking time from the right, they rise, lifting the stretcher, and face one another, place the handles of the poles between their thighs, runners to the right, *i.e.*, left of No. 1 and right of No. 3, and roll the canvas tightly over the poles to the right of the stretcher.

Taking time from the right, Nos. 1 and 3 take up a sling, and pass the grip-plate buckle) end to each other; each holds in the left hand the grip-plate end given him, threads the transverse strap through the loop of the other sling, and buckles tightly close to the roller, keeping the slings on top: then grasping both handles in their right hands, back of the hands to the right, they turn to the right in a slightly stooping position, rise, and turn to the left together. The bearers on the right (No. 4) of the stretchers now take a side pace of 30 inches (or two side paces of 15 inches) to the left. This brings No. 4 close to the stretcher.

When an injured person is picked up by a stretcher squad the procedure is as follows:—

The squad doubles by the shortest route to the injured person and halts, about a pace from the head of, and in line with, the patient. The No. 4 bearer, who is always commander of the squad, gives the order "Lower Stretcher—Prepare Stretcher."

Whilst the stretcher is being prepared by Nos. 1 and 3, the disengaged bearers proceed to the patient to render such assistance as may be required, the No. 2 going to the left, and No. 4 to the right. No. 4 may call upon Nos. 1 and 3 bearers also to assist in rendering First Aid if there are several wounds requiring immediate attention.

"*Load Stretcher.*"—When the patient is ready for removal on the stretcher, No. 4 gives the command "Load Stretcher," when the bearers place themselves as follows :—Nos. 1, 2 and 3 on the left of the patient, No. 4 on the right, No. 1 at the knees, No. 2 at the hips, No. 3 at the shoulders, No. 4 on the patient's right, opposite No. 2.

The whole turn towards the patient and kneel on the left knee, pass their hands beneath the patient ; No. 1 supports the legs, No. 2 the thighs and hips, No. 3 the upper part of the trunk, No. 4 on the right assisting to lift the patient by passing his hands beneath in corresponding position to No. 2. In lifting the patient off the ground special care must be taken of the injured part, No. 4 giving the necessary instructions for carrying out this precaution,

In the case of severe injury, No. 4 attends to the injured part in lifting.

"*Lift.*"—The No. 4 now gives the command "Lift," when the patient is carefully lifted on to the knees of Nos. 1, 2 and 3. No. 4 on the right of the patient disengages, rises, and steps back one pace: turns to his left, doubles to the stretcher, takes hold of it, left hand across, rises, the near pole resting on the left hip, returns to the patient and places it directly beneath him, then stands up. No. 4 now kneels on his left knee and assists in lowering the patient.

"*Lower.*"—The No. 4 gives the command "Lower," the patient is lowered slowly and gently on to the centre of the canvas, special care being taken of the injured part.

When the patient is laid on the stretcher, the bearers disengage, rise, Nos. 1, 2 and 3 turn to the left, No. 4 to the right, and the whole stand to stretcher as in prepared stretchers.

Unloading.

"*Unload Stretchers.*"—The bearers place themselves as described for loading, Nos. 1, 2, 3 on the left, and No. 4 on the right poposite No. 2.

If on the march, No. 4 gives the command, "Halt—Lower Stretcher—Unload Stretcher."

"*Lift.*"—The patient is lifted, as described for loading, on to the knees of Nos. 1, 2 and 3, assisted by No. 4; then No. 4 on the right of the patient disengages, rises, steps back one pace, grasps the stretcher as described for loading, and, lifting it clear of the patient, carries it forward three paces clear of the patient's feet.

He then rejoins his squad, and with the other bearers assists in lowering the patient to the ground.

"*Lower.*"—On the word "Lower," the patient is gently lowered to the ground, the bearers disengage, rise, and turn towards the stretcher, the whole stepping off to their places at the stretcher as in prepared stretchers. On completion of this exercise the stretchers are closed and the squads join their section.

The drill laid down in the Home text-book differs materially from the military drill as detailed above.

It is arranged in five exercises, but the fifth of these is for six bearers and quite unsuited for civil work.

METHOD No. 1.

For Four Bearers.

1. The instructor selects the bearers and numbers them—1, 2, 3 and 4 at his discretion. Should one man be taller and stronger than the others, he should be styled No. 3 and as he will have to bear the heavier part of the burden, all orders will be given by No. 4.

Note.—Bearers should, however, be taught to take any of the positions named in the following exercises, whether that of No. 1 2, 3 or 4 bearer.

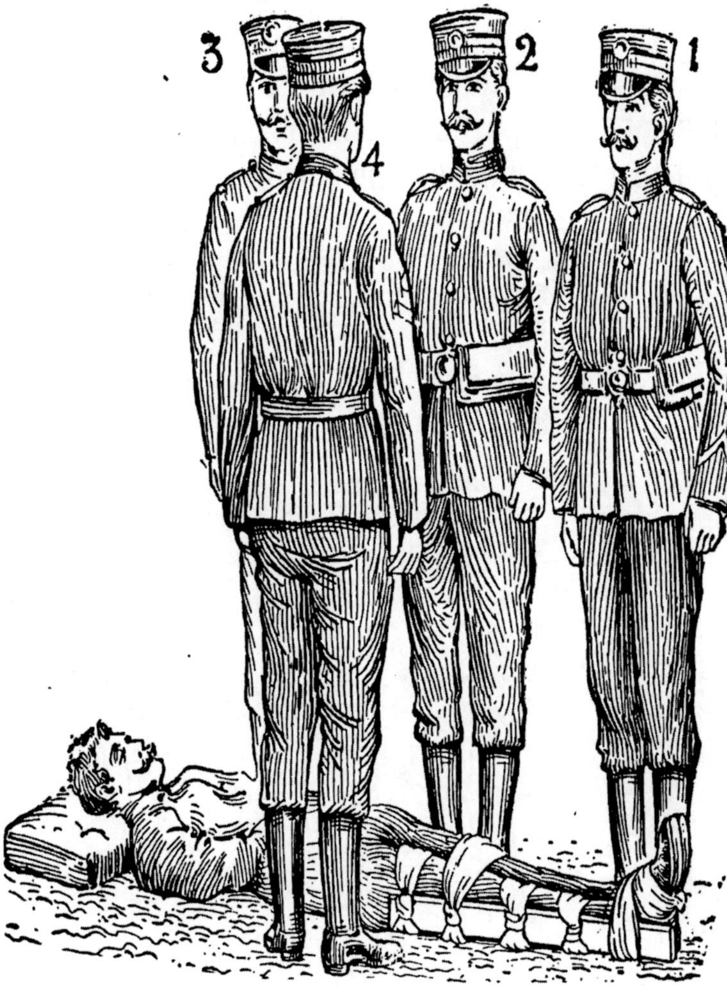

FIG. 60.

STRETCHER—EXERCISE NO. 1. FALL IN.

2. "*Fall In.*"—Nos. 1, 2 and 3 take position on the left side of and facing the patient. No. 1 places himself at the patient's knees, No. 2 at the hips, No. 3 at the patient's shoulders. At the same time No. 4 places the prepared stretcher on the ground by the right side of the patient about two

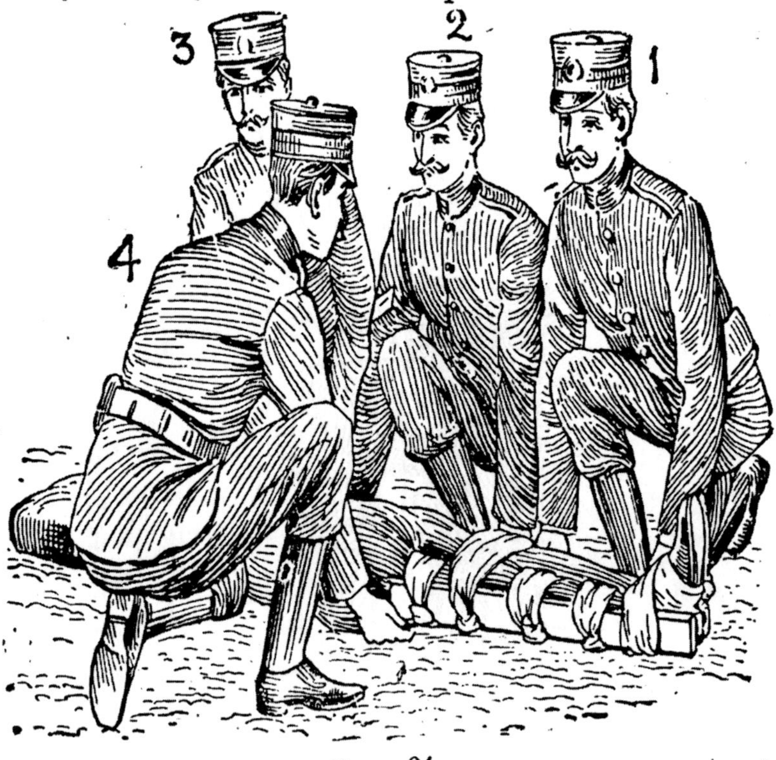

Fig. 61
STRETCHER—EXERCISE No. 1—READY TO LIFT PATIENT.

paces away from him, and then takes position opposite to and facing No. 2 (Fig. 60).

3. "*Ready.*"—The bearers kneel down on the left knee and take hold of the patient.

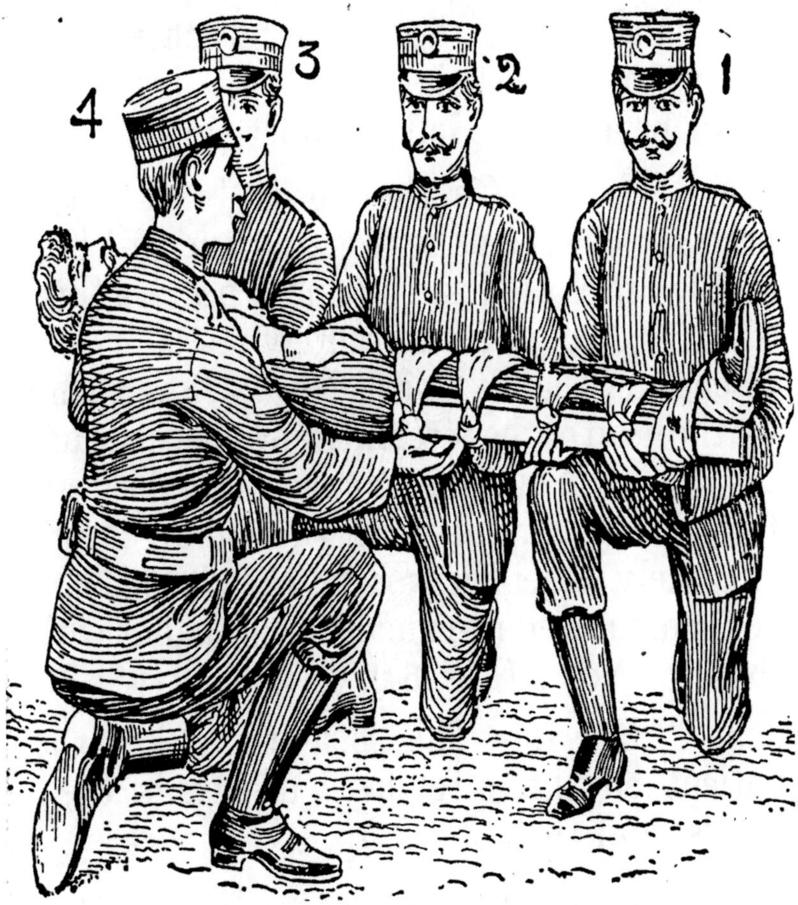

FIG. 62.

STRETCHER—EXERCISE No. 1—LIFTING PATIENT.

No. 1 passes his hands and forearms beneath the patient's legs, hands wide apart, Nos. 2 and 4 pass their hands and forearms beneath the patient's hips and loins, and grasp each other's hand. No. 3 passes his left hand across the patient's chest and under the right shoulder, and his right hand beneath the left shoulder (Fig. 61).

4. "*Lift.*"—On the word "Lift" the bearers raise the patient gently and rest him on the knees of Nos. 1, 2 and 3 bearers (Fig. 62); as soon as he is securely rested, No. 4 disengages hands with No. 2, runs round by the head of the stretcher and places it under the patient, close to the other bearers' feet, being careful that the pillow is immediately under the patient's head (Fig. 63); he then kneels down and locks his hands with those of No. 2 (Fig. 64).

5. "*Lower.*"—The bearers place the patient on the stretcher, disengage their hands, and then stand up.

6. "*Stand to Stretcher.*"—No. 1 goes to the foot of the stretcher, with his back to the patient; No. 3 to the head with his face

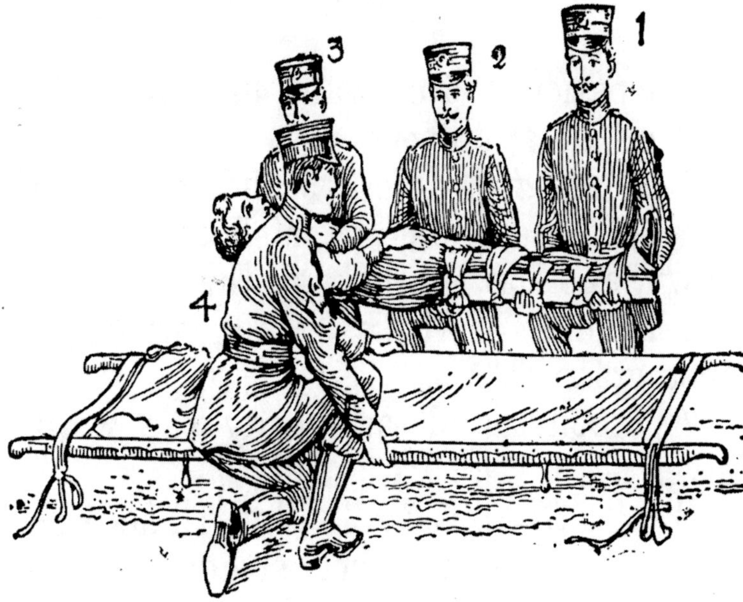

FIG. 63

STRETCHER—EXERCISE NO. 1—PLACING PATIENT.

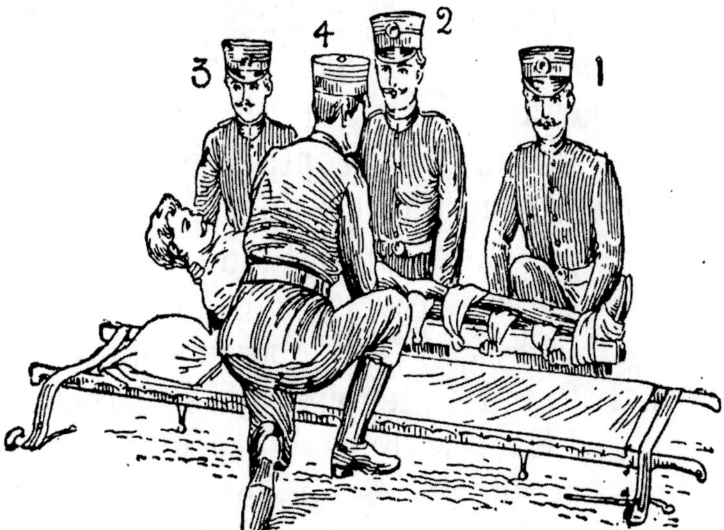

FIG. 64

STRETCHER—EXERCISE NO. 1—LOWERING PATIENT.

to the patient: Nos. 2 and 4 remain on each side of the stretcher.

7. "*Ready.*"—Nos. 1 and 3 place the slings (if used) over their shoulders, stoop down, and slip the loops of the slings on to the handles of the stretcher, which they then grasp.

As soon as all are ready the word is given:—

8. "*Lift Stretcher.*"—Nos. 1 and 3 bearers raise the stretcher steadily together and stand up.

Note.—Nos. 2 and 4 will now adjust the slings on the shoulders of Nos. 1 and 3, taking care that each is well below the level of the collar and lies accurately in the hollow of the shoulder in front. They will also lengthen or shorten the slings, having regard to the patient's injuries and the relative heights of the bearers.

9. "*March.*"—The bearers move off, Nos. 1, 2 and 4 stepping off with their left foot, and No. 3 with his right foot. (Fig. 65.) The step should be a short one of 20 inches, and taken with bent knees and no spring from the fore part of the foot.

10. "*Halt.*"—The bearers remain steady.

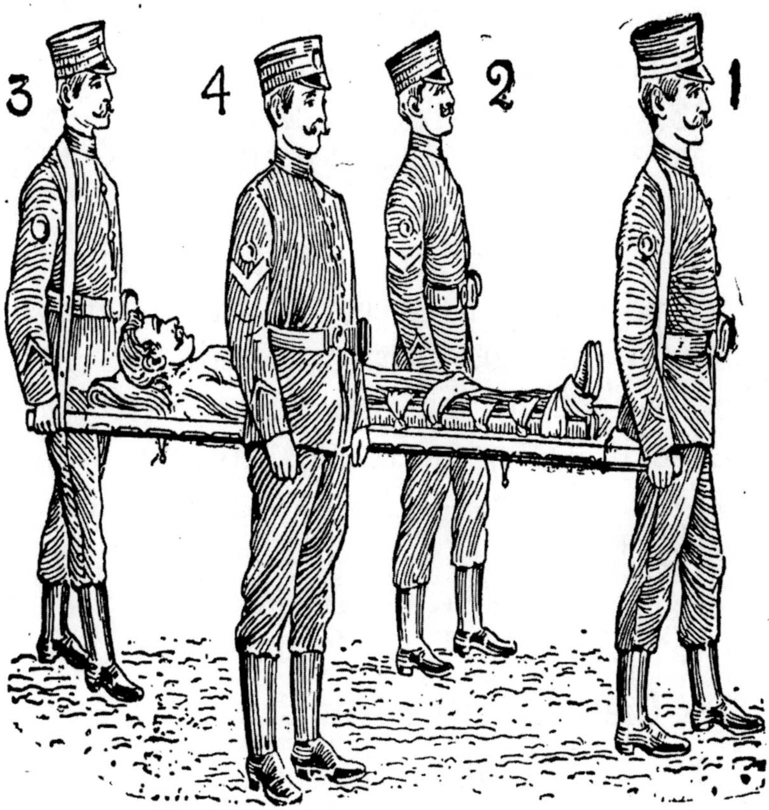

FIG. 65

STRETCHER—EXERCISE No. 1—MARCH.

11. "*Lower Stretcher.*"—The bearers place the stretcher gently on the ground, slip the loops in the slings off the handles of the stretcher, remove the slings from the shoulders and then stand up.

12. "*Unload Stretcher—Ready.*"—The bearers prepare to take the patient off stretcher as at orders 2 and 3.

13. "*Lift.*"—The bearers raise the patient as at order 4 (Fig. 64); No. 4, in this case, disengages hands from No. 2, removes the stretcher, and resumes his former position. If necessary, the bearers will steadily rise together, and carefully carry the patient to the bed, or other place to which it has been arranged to convey him.

14. "*Lower.*"—The patient is carefully lowered.

METHOD No. 2.
For Three Bearers.

(The Bearers are Numbered 1, 2, 3.)

The squad is under the command of No. 2. The stretcher is placed in line with the patient's body quite close to his head.

The patient is raised by the three bearers and carried over the foot of the stretcher until his head is in line with the pillow. He is carefully lowered on to the stretcher bed. Nos. 1 and 3 then lift and carry the stretcher and No. 2 looks after the patient.

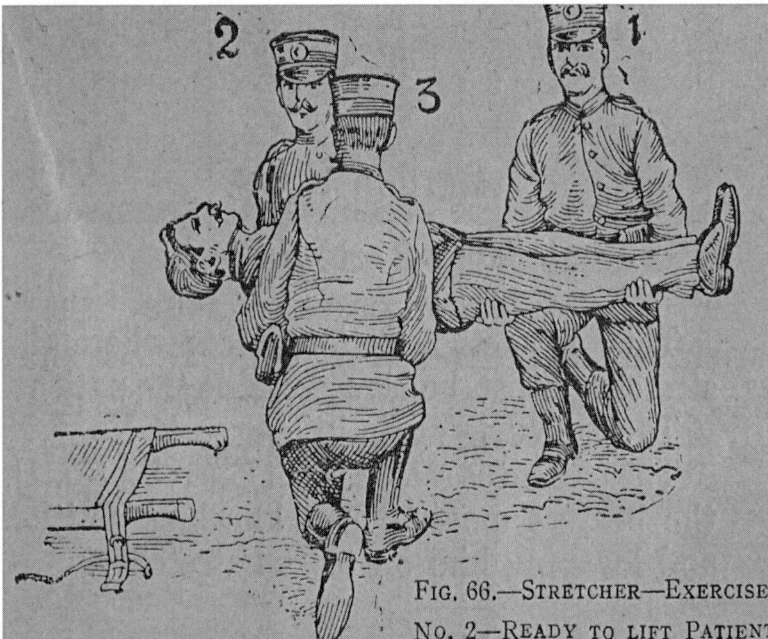

FIG. 66.—STRETCHER—EXERCISE NO. 2—READY TO LIFT PATIENT.

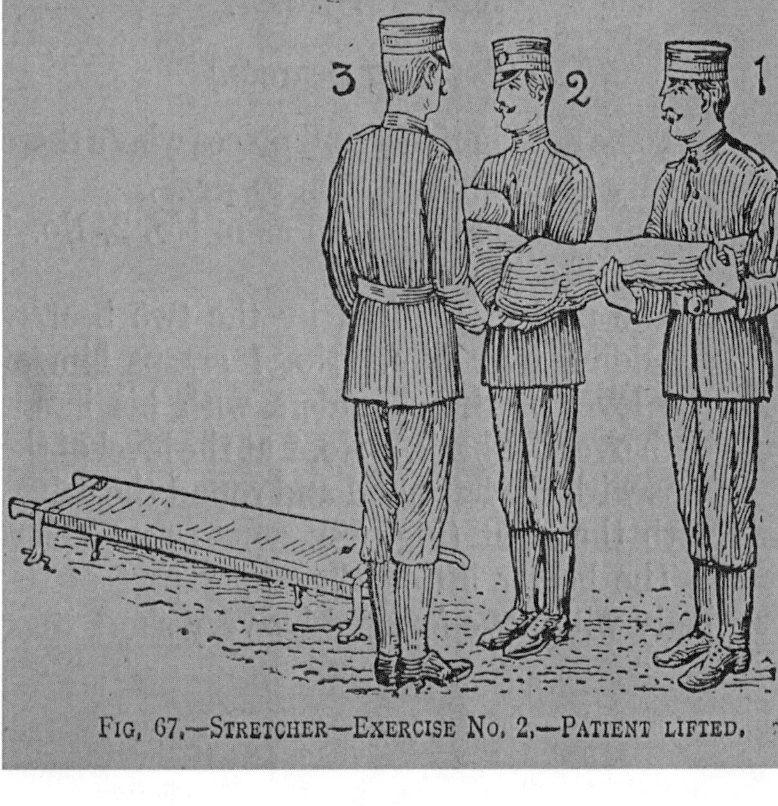

FIG, 67.—STRETCHER—EXERCISE NO. 2.—PATIENT LIFTED.

Method No. 3.

(Also for Three Bearers.)

This is designed for places where the stretcher must be placed beside the patient.

The squad is again in charge of No. 2.

The patient is raised (as in Exercise No. 1), the bearers moving in a kneeling position and lowering him on to the stretcher.

Method No. 4.

(For Two Bearers.)

To be used in mines and places where there is only room for two men to work.

The stretcher is placed as in No. 2, No. 1 is the directing bearer.

The patient is lifted by the two bearers straddling over him. No. 1 grasps him at the level of the shoulders with his hands both over the back. No. 2 at the level of the hips with the left hand and round the calves with the right (Fig. 68).

The bearer lifting the upper part of the body will move forward by very short steps and the other will bend his body forward as much as he can without moving his feet.

No. 1 now orders No. 2 to halt and remain steady whilst he advances his right foot to his left, and then his left until his toe touches the heel of No. 2.

These movements are repeated until the patient can be lowered on to the stretcher (Fig. 69).

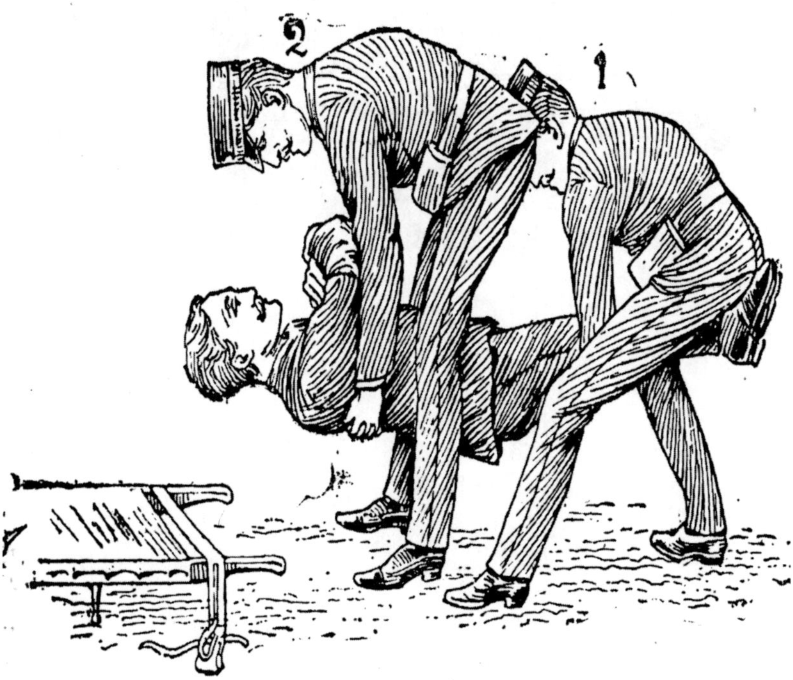

FIG. 68

STRETCHER—EXERCISE NO. 4—FIRST POSITION.

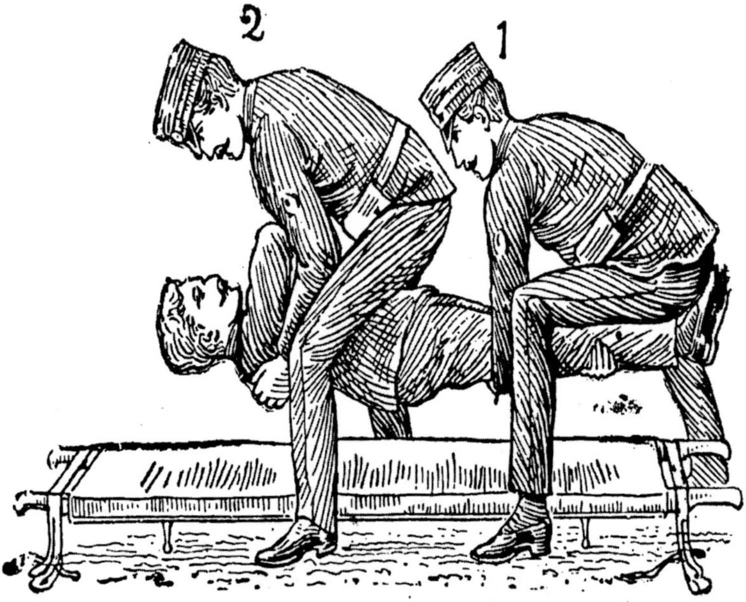

FIG. 69

STRETCHER—EXERCISE NO. 4—SECOND POSITION.

CHAPTER XVII.

Home Arrangements for Accidents and Emergencies.

The following points have to be considered :—

1. The preparation of the room.
2. The lifting and carrying of the sick or injured person.
3. The preparation of the bed.
4. The removal of the clothes.
5. The preparation for the doctor.

1. *The preparation of the room.*—Often there can be no choice of a sick-room.

If possible it should be :—

1. A sunny room.
2. A quiet room.
3. A large room.

A sunny room is far more healthy than a dark one and quite as cool. The popular delusion that a dark room is cooler than one into which indirect sunlight enters freely dies hard in India. The first gift that God gave the world was light, and it is the greatest. Light and life, death and darkness go together.

2. *The Lifting and Carrying of the Sick or Unjured Person.*—This subject is fully dealt with in Chapter XVI. Under the St. John Ambulance rules, women are not taught stretcher drill, but the Red Cross Training Manual says :—" Women ought to learn stretcher drill. Should a woman be in a country district with no available help except untrained country folk, it is expedient to be able to direct how a wounded man should be lifted, how an improvised stretcher can be put together, and how the stretcher should be carried. Women should not be allowed to carry wounded men on stretchers, unless there are six women bearers, one at each end of the stretcher, and four more supporting the sides of the stretcher."

3. *The Preparation of the Bed.*—The best kind of bed for a long illness is a single size iron bedstead, with a woven wire mattress, and one coir or wool mattress over that. Such beds are, however, not suitable for fractures of the thigh or leg. In these cases, where a special fracture bed is not available, the bed can be made sufficiently rigid by placing a board over the wire mattress and beneath the coir one.

A mattress case filled with fresh clean straw is very good for people who can afford no better. It can be emptied out and refilled at trifling cost. In the sick-room nothing should be kept under the bed. The common Indian habit of keeping boxes, bundles, and lumber of all sorts under the bed is bad at any time. It is most objectionable in illness, when air is particularly wanted under the bed to keep it pure.

A patient can be much more easily nursed in a bed that is not too large. If practicable it is very desirable to have two small beds, so that the patient can be moved from one to the other occasionally.

The sick-bed should never be placed with one side against the wall as the nurse must be able to get at both sides of the bed.

For accident cases the mattress should always be covered with some waterproof material. Waterproof sheeting is the best covering, but is most expensive. American cloth, such as is sometimes used to cover washstands, is a substitute readily obtainable in India.

In arranging the sheets on the sick-bed, care must be taken to prevent the under-sheet from becoming crumpled under the patient. This can be prevented by pulling the sheet quite smooth over the bed, tucking it in tightly under the mattress, and then firmly pinning it to the underside of the bed with several strong safety-pins.

A draw-sheet saves the under-sheet from frequent changing, and keeps the bed clean and comfortable. It is arranged as follows :—Fold the sheet in two, *lengthways*, roll up one end until there is just enough of the folded sheet left to reach across the bed. The roll is tucked under the mattress, and firmly pinned in place ; the rest is laid over the under-sheet across the bed, just where the middle of the patient's body lies, and is firmly pinned under the mattress on the side opposite to the rolled part. If the part under the patient becomes damp, slightly soiled or hot (which in fever it often does), instead of having to change the entire under-sheet it is only necessary to unpin the draw-sheet, take the end *opposite the rolled part* and draw under the patient a clean dry piece, roll up, tuck under, and pin as before.

A strip of waterproof material should also be laid *over* the under-sheet beneath the draw-sheet and pinned firmly to prevent creases.

In fractures of the lower limb some means of keeping the weight of the bed clothes off the injured part should be devised. An empty whisky or wine box with the ends taken away or a kerosine oil tin with the top and bottom and one side removed are articles always obtainable in India well adapted for use as cradles (Fig. 70).

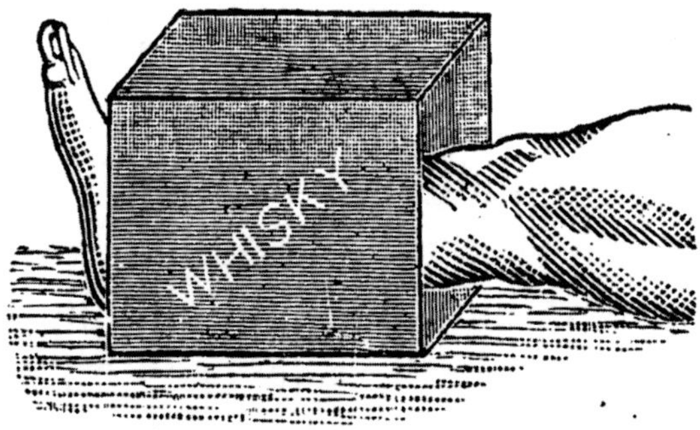

FIG. 70.—IMPROVISED BED CRADLE.

To help patients to raise themselves, or to alter their position in bed, fasten a strap with a loop, or a long roller towel to the end of the bed, and leave it on the counterpane within reach of the hand.

4. *Removal of Clothes.*—Before putting the patient in bed the clothes should be removed, and great care should be taken in doing this. In serious cases it is better to remove the clothes by cutting them away.

In removing a coat from an injured arm, draw out the uninjured arm first, and in putting on anything put the injured arm in first. In removing trousers from an injured limb, rip up the outside seam.

In removing clothes in cases of burns and scalds, cut away the parts which are not adhering, and soak the adhering parts well in boracic or carbolic lotion or warm oil, before removing them.

5. *The Preparation for the Doctor.*—When sending for medical help, *always send a written statement* as to what the patient is suffering from. If this is done, the doctor will bring with him the appliances and remedies likely to be required. This saves much time and in many accidents may actually save life. Ten minutes delay, for instance, in hæmorrhage or poisoning, make all the difference to the prospects of saving the patient's life.

In cases of all severe injuries the following should be got ready for the surgeon's visit :—

(1) Plenty of hot and cold water.
(2) Clean towels and soap.
(3) A nail brush.
(4) Nail scissors, and
(5) A slop bucket.

The following articles should be obtained if possible for the treatment of special injuries :—

(*A*). *For Burns and Scalds* :—

(1) Plenty of lint.
(2) Absorbent cotton wool.
(3) Olive oil.
(4) Vaseline with eucalyptus oil (thirty drops) added to each ounce.
(5) Carbolic lotion (1 in 20).
(6) Bandages, and
(7) Boric powder.

(*B*). *For Hæmorrhage* :—

Ice and sponges or swabs of absorbent cotton wool.

(*C*). *For Drowning* :—

(1) Several blankets warmed before the fire.
(2) Hot tea and coffee.
(3) Brandy or whisky and sal volatile.
(4) Hot-water bottles, and
(5) Remove the sheets from the bed.

(*D*). *For open Wounds of any kind :—*

(1) Tincture of Iodine.
(2) Boric lint.
(3) Swabs of absorbent cotton wool.
(4) Boric lotion.
(5) Soloids of Perchloride of Mercury.
(6) Gutta-percha tissue or oiled silk.
(7) Several bandages.
(8) A pair of scissors.
(9) Safety pins.
(10) A pair of dressing forceps (if possible).

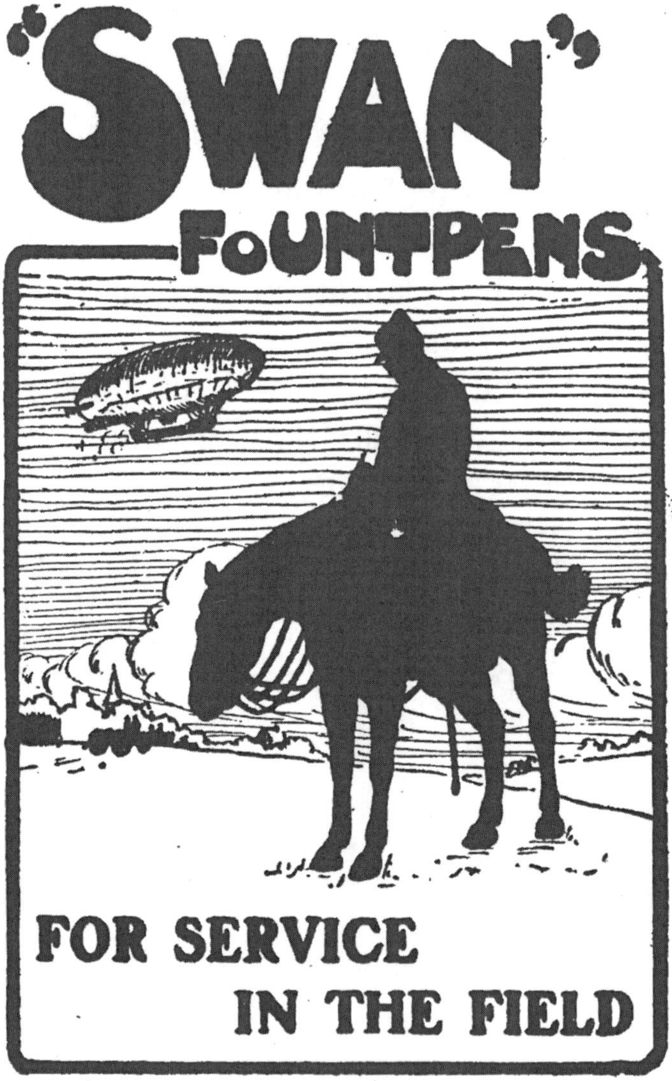

All grades of Swan Pens at London Prices,
Can be had from

WHITEAWAY, LAIDLAW & Co., Ld.,
BOMBAY.

INDEX.

A

B

C

D

E

F

G

H

I

J

K

L

R

S

W

LEACH & WEBORNY,

Naval and Military Tailors,

BOMBAY, POONA & BUSRA.

Before placing your order for Uniforms and Camp Furniture, etc., consult the above named firm, who are Specialists in this work and guarantee satisfaction.

EVANS, FRASER & Co.,

BOMBAY.

BRANCH AT BASRAH, PERSIAN GULF.

GENERAL DRAPERS AND OUTFITTERS, FURNISHERS, IMPORTERS OF BOOTS AND SHOES, HARDWARE, GLASSWARE, Etc., GOVERNMENT CONTRACTORS.

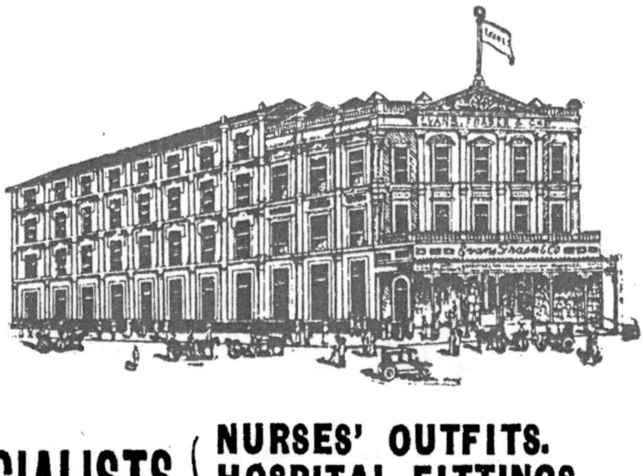

SPECIALISTS IN
- **NURSES' OUTFITS.**
- **HOSPITAL FITTINGS.**
- **CAMP OUTFITS.**
- **OFFICERS' SERVICE REQUIREMENTS.**

A large General Illustrated Catalogue will be sent free to any address in India, Burmah, Ceylon or Mesopotamia by return of post free of charge.

Nurses interested in Art Needlework should write for a copy of our Smallwares Catalogue, which is also sent free. It contains a marvellous collection of Smallwares and Art Needlework Goods and also much useful information.

WRITE TO-DAY AND GET INTO TOUCH WITH US.